The Claustro-Agoraphobic Dilemma in Psychoanalysis

This collection addresses the theory of claustro-agoraphobic anxieties and schizoid phenomena. It provides psychoanalytic case studies of the transference and counter-transference dynamic inherent in these agonizing disorders.

In *The Claustro-Agoraphobic Dilemma in Psychoanalysis: Fear of Madness*, Susan Finkelstein and Heinz Weiss gather both classic papers and new essays, presenting a timely assessment of claustro-agoraphobia as first developed by Henri Rey. This volume includes papers by Helene Deutsch, Bertram Lewin, Edoardo Weiss, Esther Bick, Donald Meltzer, Albert Mason, John Steiner, and Claudia Frank, as well as a chapter by Kristin White on working remotely with psychoanalytic patients during the Covid-19 pandemic. Applying a Freudian, Kleinian, and Bionian methodology, this collection argues for a long-term approach to psychoanalytic treatment in order to help claustro-agoraphobic patients work through the unconscious conflicts that interfere with their capacity to engage in a committed relationship.

This book is essential reading for psychoanalysts in practice and training and will appeal to academics and historians interested in the universality of spiritual and mythic motifs.

Susan Finkelstein is Faculty Member and Training and Supervising Analyst at the Contemporary Freudian Society and the Institute for Psychoanalytic Training and Research. She is Director of Understanding Primitive Mental States and an associate board member of the *International Journal of Psychoanalysis*. She practices psychoanalysis, supervision, and couples therapy in New York City.

Heinz Weiss, MD, is Head of the Department of Psychosomatic Medicine at the Robert-Bosch-Clinic, Stuttgart, Germany, Head of the Medical Department, and Member of the Directorate of the Sigmund Freud-Institute, Frankfurt, Germany. He teaches at the University of Tübingen and chairs the Education Section of the *International Journal of Psychoanalysis*.

'This book was in a sense waiting to be produced. I say this because the phenomenon of claustro-agoraphobia is a core dimension of the human condition and, though not always recognized as such, enters the consulting room with every patient. It is a concept we use every day without necessarily naming it or understanding its theoretical and historical significance. In *Group Psychology and the Analysis of the Ego*, Freud quoted Schopenhauer on the "hedgehogs' dilemma". In my paraphrasing, hedgehogs huddle together in winter to get warm, but when they get too close, they prick each other and move apart. But then they feel cold and huddle together again. And so, they spend the whole winter moving together and apart, trying to find a place where they can be near enough to get warm but not so near that they get hurt – the poetic evocation of a universal human dilemma.

All forms of psychopathology, then, have a claustro-agoraphobic dimension. Patients feel trapped with their symptoms and the objects that persecute them – their marriages, their jobs, their relationships, but more than anything with the contents of their own minds.

The editors have provided us with a superb selection of papers ranging from Helene Deutsch's 1929 essay to works that are part of our contemporary psychoanalytic world (Rey, Meltzer, Steiner) and that deepen and broaden our understanding of this concept both in terms of its clinical phenomenology and its theoretical underpinnings. The editors' Introduction provides a rich cultural perspective and mapping out of the concepts. The editors also provide historical links to ancient philosophy and the world of literature.

This is a book that all clinicians – psychologists, psychiatrists, and psychoanalysts – will find fascinating and enriching. *The Claustro-Agoraphobic Dilemma in Psychoanalysis: Fear of Madness* will find its place as a key text. A must for all libraries.'

David Bell, *BSc, MB, MRCP, FRCPsych, Psychoanalyst;*
Former President of the British Psychoanalytical Society;
Former Consultant Psychiatrist at Tavistock Clinic, UK

'Susan Finkelstein and Heinz Weiss have thoughtfully compiled many of the most significant theoretical and clinical papers on the fascinating and important topic of the claustro-agoraphobic dilemma. The collection of papers, from Lewin's to Steiner's on Psychic Retreat, from Henri Rey's to Meltzer's ideas on the Claustrum, covers both historical contributions and theoretical differences. Readers are also treated to original chapters by the editors and contributors that place the more historical papers within a modern context. The introduction to the book and the prefaces provide clear, erudite, and concise statements of the central ideas for each chapter. This is an excellent and invaluable addition to any psychotherapist's or psychoanalyst's library.'

Abbot A. Bronstein, *PhD, Editor of* The Analyst at Work *and the*
International Journal of Psychology; *Psychoanalyst; Chair of the North*
American Comparative Clinical Methods Working Party Group; Former IPA
Board Member and TA/SA at the San Francisco Center of Psychoanalysis, USA

'Claustro-agoraphobia constitutes the natural dilemma of those who have not developed a true personality. These people are always afraid of being trapped and dominated in the interpersonal relationship that they escape to find themselves in the anguish of emptiness. This book reports the most useful psychoanalytic contributions on the subject and opens new perspectives to this still unsolved aspect of the psyche. A commendable and useful contribution to bring psychoanalysis back to clinical research.'

Franco de Masi, *Training and Supervising Analyst of the Italian Psychoanalytical Society; Former President of Centro Milanese di Psicoanalisi and Secretary of the Training Milanese Institute, Italy*

'This book not only offers many interesting reflections on the psychoanalytic concept of claustro-agoraphobia but, in fact, establishes its meaning and value. It shows how a range of different clinical phenomena and dynamics discussed in the analytic literature, past and present, share dimensions which allow them to be more deeply understood when brought together under the notion of claustro-agoraphobia.'

Rachel Blass, *Training Analyst at the Israel Psychoanalytic Society and Member of the British Psychoanalytical Society, UK*

The Claustro-Agoraphobic Dilemma in Psychoanalysis

Fear of Madness

Edited by Susan Finkelstein and Heinz Weiss

Routledge
Taylor & Francis Group

LONDON AND NEW YORK

Cover image: Piranesi, Giovanni Battista. *The Round Tower from Carceri d'invenzione*, 1749–1750. The Metropolitan Museum of Art. Harris Brisbane Dick Fund, 1937. www.metmuseum.org

First published 2023
by Routledge
4 Park Square, Milton Park, Abingdon, Oxon OX14 4RN

and by Routledge
605 Third Avenue, New York, NY 10158

Routledge is an imprint of the Taylor & Francis Group, an informa business

British Library Cataloguing-in-Publication Data
A catalogue record for this book is available from the British Library

Library of Congress Cataloging-in-Publication Data
Names: Finkelstein, Susan, editor. | Weiss, Heinz, 1955- editor.
Title: The claustro-agoraphobic dilemma in psychoanalysis: fear of madness / edited by Susan Finkelstein and Heinz Weiss.
Description: New York, NY: Routledge, 2023. | Identifiers: LCCN 2022021183 (print) | LCCN 2022021184 (ebook) | ISBN 9781032060149 (paperback) | ISBN 9781032060132 (hardback) | ISBN 9781003200284 (ebook)
Subjects: LCSH: Psychoanalysis. | Claustrophobia. | Agoraphobia. | Schizoid personality.
Classification: LCC RC506 .C525 2023 (print) | LCC RC506 (ebook) | DDC 616.89/17—dc23/eng/20220816
LC record available at https://lccn.loc.gov/2022021183
LC ebook record available at https://lccn.loc.gov/2022021184

ISBN: 978-1-032-06013-2 (hbk)
ISBN: 978-1-032-06014-9 (pbk)
ISBN: 978-1-003-20028-4 (ebk)

DOI: 10.4324/9781003200284

Typeset in Times New Roman
by Apex CoVantage, LLC

Contents

Contributors

Susan Finkelstein is a faculty member and training and supervising analyst at the Contemporary Freudian Society and the Institute for Research and Psychoanalytic Training (IPTAR), both in NYC. She is an associate editor of the *International Journal of Psychoanalysis* and the director of Understanding Primitive Mental States, a program of international study groups on Klein, Bion, and the British Independent Tradition. She practices psychoanalysis, psychotherapy, and couples therapy in NYC.

Claudia Frank, Priv.-Doz. Dr. Med., is a psychoanalyst in private practice in Stuttgart, Germany, and a training analyst of the DPV/IPA. She spent 1988–2001 at the Department for Psychoanalysis, Psychotherapy, and Psychosomatics at the University of Tübingen. She is a guest member of the British Psychoanalytical Society. From 2016 to 2018, she was the chair of the Central Training Committee of the DPV. Her research focuses on the history, technique, and theory of Kleinian analysis with various publications, such as *Melanie Klein in Berlin: Her First Psychoanalyses of Children* (2009, Routledge) and a paper with J. Milton (ed.), *Essential Readings from the Melanie Klein Archives* (2020, Routledge), next to papers in applied psychoanalysis (psychosomatics; on Antigone; Giacometti, Morandi, etc.). She was a co-editor of *Jahrbuch der Psychoanalyse* from 2002 to 2013. Together with Heinz Weiß, she is the editor of various books on Kleinian psychoanalysis in German.

John Steiner is a training analyst of the British Psychoanalytical Society and was formerly a psychiatrist at the Maudsley Hospital and a psychotherapist at the Tavistock Clinic. He has now retired from clinical practice but continues to supervise and write. He is the author of *Psychic Retreats* (1993), *Seeing and Being Seen* (2011), and *Illusion, Disillusion and Irony in Psychoanalysis* (2020). He has also edited and written introductions to *The Oedipus Complex Today* (1989), *Psychoanalysis, Literature and War* (Hanna Segal, 1997), *Rosenfeld in Retrospect* (2008), and Melanie Klein's 1936 *Lectures on Technique* (2017).

Heinz Weiss is the head of the Department of Psychosomatic Medicine, Robert-Bosch-Hospital Stuttgart; the head of the Medical Division and a member of the Directorate, Sigmund-Freud-Institute, Frankfurt/Main; a professor at the University of Tubingen; and the chair of the Education Section of the *International Journal of Psychoanalysis*, Germany.

Kristin White, Dipl.-Psych., is a psychoanalyst working with adults and children in English and German, with a practice in the centre of Berlin, Germany. She is also a training analyst, lecturer, and clinical supervisor at the Alfred-Adler Training Institute for Psychoanalysis and Psychotherapy in Berlin. She is a training member of the German Society for Psychoanalysis and Psychotherapy (DGPT) and the German Adlerian Society (DGIP). Until 2021, she was a member of the editing team of the *Zeitschrift für Individualpsychologie*, an Adlerian journal for psychoanalysis, psychotherapy, and counselling and has published a number of papers in this journal in German. She is a member of the board of reviewers for the *International Journal of Psychoanalysis* and has also written papers for this journal in English. Her writing has focused particularly on the topic of migration and psychoanalysis, which is also the central theme of the book *Migration and Intercultural Psychoanalysis*, edited by Kristin White and Ina Klingenberg and published by Routledge in 2020.

Acknowledgements

The publication of this volume was possible only with the help of many colleagues and institutions who have contributed to our personal and professional lives.

We affectionately acknowledge John Steiner for his shared passion for Henri Rey and for his foreword and support of the publication of this book.

Our families have contributed to our emotional and intellectual development in countless ways.

Our patients have shared their souls and minds with us, for which we are grateful. Our many students, supervisees, and colleagues, particularly those studying with us in our Understanding Primitive Mental States clinical and theoretical seminar on claustro-agoraphobia, have enriched our understanding of the psychoanalytic concepts depicted in this book.

Routledge and its general editor, Susannah Frearson, provided advice and encouragement from start to finish. Emily Steadman secured copyright permissions.

We would like to thank the *International Journal of Psychoanalysis* for permission to reprint the papers by Helene Deutsch, Donald Meltzer, Edoardo Weiss, and Heinz Weiss. *The British Journal of Psychotherapy* gave permission to reprint the paper by Esther Bick. *The Psychoanalytic Quarterly* granted permission to reprint the paper by Bertram Lewin. We are grateful to Routledge for permitting the republication of papers by Albert Mason and John Steiner. Despite extensive research, we were unable to locate the copyright for the paper by Henri Rey (Rey, H. (1994); *Universals of psychoanalysis in the treatment of psychotic and borderline states*; Magagna, J. (ed.); London: Free Association Books; Chapter 2, pp. 8–31). All efforts have been made to trace the copyright holders of material in this book. Any omissions brought to the attention of the publisher will be rectified in a subsequent edition.

We gratefully acknowledge the Metropolitan Museum of Art Collection, New York City, and its open-access policy that allows the reprint of this Piranesi etching on our front cover.

Furthermore, we are pleased to thank colleagues and friends whose generous advice was indispensable in our pursuit of this project, in particular David Bell, Dana Birksted-Breen, Ronald Britton, Irma Brenman Pick, Michael Feldman, Lynne Herbst, Edna O'Shaughnessy, and Enid Stubin. We are grateful for their help and support, and we hope that the publication of this volume will further stimulate interest in this fascinating area of mental life.

Foreword

John Steiner

Claustrophobia and agoraphobia are common conditions, and the relationship between them, described by Henri Rey as the claustro-agoraphobic dilemma, helps us understand that, in many patients, they coexist. The patient tries to find safety by coming close to his object, often with phantasies of getting inside them, but then becomes anxious, feels trapped, and tries to escape. Once outside, he feels unprotected, and becoming anxious again, he tries to get back inside. This means that there is nowhere that the patient feels safe and no identity that he feels comfortable with. This situation was described by Henri Rey, a French-speaking psychoanalyst from the island of Mauritius who spent his professional life at the Maudsley Hospital, where he introduced psychoanalytic ideas and influenced a generation of young analysts, including me. His wonderfully lively teaching style and the originality of his ideas do not always emerge in his rather sparse writings, and his papers are often quite muddled and difficult to understand. Nevertheless, his exploration of spatial models of the mind is of fundamental importance in helping us to understand claustro-agoraphobia on the one hand and object relationships in general on the other. One of the great virtues of this book is introducing the work of Henri Rey to a wider audience.

His exploration of the three-dimensional world of object relations helps us to understand the infantile needs and fears that give rise to anxiety. Furthermore, he has shown how the concrete nature of internal objects in borderline and psychotic patients, which accentuates anxiety and makes escape difficult. Heinz Weiss has explored this theme in an earlier volume (Weiss 2020), in which he describes what he calls the Joan Riviere dilemma, in which the individual can neither repair nor escape from the persecuting demands of his damaged internal objects. Joan Riviere was one of Henri Rey's supervisors, and it is his understanding of the enormous advantages of symbolic reparation that has allowed us to understand the plight of many patients trapped in a world of concrete objects.[1]

Rey describes early object relations with a maternal object characterised by an external boundary and an internal space which is commonly idealised to form a Garden of Eden which promises bliss without end and is associated with the inside of the mother's body. When the idealisation breaks down, two kinds of phantasies are involved. In the first, which is associated with claustrophobia, the maternal space turns out to be occupied by rivals that threaten the intruder in terrifying primitive part-object phantasies. Here the patient discovers that the mother contains frightening persecutors, often taking the form of her unborn babies and the father's penis, and these transform her body from the idealised haven he expects into a persecuting space from which he is desperate to escape.

At other times, and this is associated with agoraphobia, the intruder manages to escape, but once outside, he feels that he has been prematurely ejected to fend for himself in an external world that is full of predators. The maternal space is once more idealised, and regaining access to it becomes the one way to relieve the anxiety.

When concrete thinking predominates, the containing mother is conceived in equally concrete terms, which Henri Rey illustrated by referring to the Maudsley Hospital as a 'Brick Mother'. This shows both the strengths and the weaknesses of a containing object which provides stability but no real understanding. Containment is provided by an exoskeleton in which the vulnerable infant can find protection in a hard shell such as that of shellfish. When the patient internalises this type of containment, he creates a composite self-object existing in both body and mind as a thing that is not able to partake in symbolic activities, such as thinking and dreaming, and hence is dealt with by projective identification. To establish symbolic function, further developments are required in which the object needs to be relinquished and mourned. The object is then internalised in a different way, no longer as a ghost but as an ancestor,[2] and a new freedom of thought is established. Rey likened this development to the development of a backbone or spinal column, which in evolution represents a huge advance, especially in the area of mobility.[3] The understanding of the importance of the ability to use symbols is especially relevant to the area of reparation, and the patient with concrete thinking feels obliged to repair his internal object concretely, omnipotently bringing them to life and magically restoring them in efforts that inevitably fail. In a beautiful paper on reparation, Rey shows how allowing personal development can repair an internal object. He used to enjoy describing a young mother who initially avoided having a family because she believed that she had to look after her dead mother. When she was eventually able to let this concrete demand go and become a good mother herself, the internal image of her mother as a good object was restored.

I have emphasised the work of Rey because, in my view, it is his ideas that are fundamental to the understanding of claustro-agoraphobia and object relations in general, but the editors of the book have collected together a variety of other papers that provides a background to the topic. The book begins with a selection of classical papers and continues with contemporary work, and the reader will find much of this of both theoretical and practical relevance.

A special mention should be made of Susan Finkelstein's chapter, which is an account of Hesiod's *Theogony* describing the old gods, the ancestors of the more familiar family residing on Mt Olympus. The primitive nature of the myths reveals a striking similarity to the primitive phantasies found by Klein in her descriptions of the primitive super-ego. They involve entering the mother's body and trapping the children found there by blocking their exit through endless intercourse, castration, cannibalism, and giving birth through the mouth by vomiting. Zeus managed to escape from this claustrophobic world and establish a new family dominated by a powerful father, perhaps illustrating the shift to a patrilineal society.

Notes

1 It is said that Riviere found that only two of the many analysts she supervised were exceptional, and these were Hanna Segal and Henri Rey.
2 Hans Loewald (1960) has a described the purpose of psychoanalysis, 'To turn ghosts into ancestors.'
3 Rey would give examples from a wonderful book describing the evolution of vertebrates, Buchsbaum, R. (1971). *Animals without Backbones*. Penguin Books.

References

Loewald, H.W. (1960). On the Therapeutic Action of Psycho-Analysis. *The International Journal of Psychoanalysis* 41: 16–33.
Rey, J.H. (1986). Reparation. *The Journal of the Melanie Klein Society* 4: 5–35.
Weiss, H. (2020 [2019]). *Trauma, Guilt and Reparation. The Path from Impasse to Development*. London and New York: Routledge; Stuttgart: Klett-Cotta.

Introduction

Heinz Weiss

'Claustro-agoraphobia' is a combined term for persons who can tolerate neither intimacy nor separateness in their personal relationships without feeling trapped, confused, or abandoned. This lifelong difficulty often repeats itself in the immediacy of the patient-analyst relationship, where the patient feels trapped, used, suffocated, annihilated, or abandoned by the analyst. A dread of psychic death can emerge during weekend and holiday breaks. Self and object differentiation can lead to a fear of being driven mad by the analyst, as well as the terror of retribution for the unconscious hostility, dependency needs, and hatred directed toward the analyst.

Destructive phantasies, both those projected and re-introjected, can take the analyst by surprise in the form of a sudden negative therapeutic reaction, resulting in an abrupt interruption of the treatment. Claustro-agoraphobic patients also have problems sharing 'space'. Distortions of inside and outside, who is who, confusion between subject and object, persecutory guilt, bizarre bodily sensations, and hypochondriacal and paranoid-schizoid infantile anxieties cause distortion in thinking and reduced capacity for reflection in the patient. The intensity of these defences and their projection into the analyst make it difficult for the analyst to think or formulate an interpretation.

The concept of the claustro-agoraphobic dilemma, while endemic to civilization, was not coined until 1979, when Henri Rey combined the separate but apposite well-known phobias of claustrophobia and agoraphobia (Rey 1994a, 1994b). Claustro-agoraphobic anxiety is commonly experienced in schizoid, narcissistic, and borderline patients but also occurs in neurotic and even in seemingly 'normal' individuals. The dilemma has far-reaching consequences on the individual's sense of identity, capacity for symbolic thinking, awareness of reality, and experience of time. Claustro-agoraphobic anxieties develop from early traumatic experiences and lack of maternal containment. Without them, the healthy construction of mental space is inhibited (Weiss 2020a).

The Claustro-Agoraphobic Dilemma in Psychoanalysis: Fear of Madness aims to inform analysts, mental health professionals, and the general health community about the theory and clinical nature of this condition, as well as its historical aetiology in psychoanalytic theory and literature. Chapters 1 through 8 include reprints of seminal historical contributions to the understanding of claustro-agoraphobia. Chapters 9 through 12 include contemporary essays and research on the technical challenges and treatment implications of working with these patients.

While familiar with the experience of working with claustro-agoraphobic patients, analysts are often unaware of the aetiology of this important psychoanalytic concept. Exploring and identifying its manifestations and origins are relevant for the practising psychoanalyst but also for medical practitioners, hospitalists, and scholars in cultural, philosophical, and literary backgrounds who want to understand conditions of isolation, aloneness, and lack of relationship.

Claustro-agoraphobia is related to the evolution of the concepts of time and space. It was Sigmund Freud who emphasized the importance of the space-time continuum for healthy psychic development. In his theory, the mental apparatus was described in spatial terms. He highlighted the distinction between external and internal reality: 'as much unknown to us as the reality of the external world, and . . . as incompletely presented to us by the data of consciousness as is the external world by the communications of our sense organs' (Freud 1900, p. 617). According to Freud, our internal world is peopled early on by unconscious phantasies, which sometimes interfere and overlap with external reality. This process can lead to distortions and confusion, giving rise to fears and phobic anxieties. Amongst these fears is 'the dread of being buried alive', which he connects to phantasies about life in the womb. He supposes that this fear, like the belief in survival after death, 'merely represents a projection into the future of this uncanny life before birth . . . Moreover, the act of birth is the prototype of the affect of anxiety' (Freud 1900, p. 400; see also Freud 1919).

Both the German word 'Angst' and the English word 'anxiety' refer to the Latin 'angustiae' (i.e. 'narrowness'), which Freud (1916–1917, p. 396) equated with the narrow space of the birth canal through which we are born. Thus, one might see this leaving of the maternal womb as the first experience of differentiation between the internal and external world.

Freud also examined other anxieties whose origins and dynamics were identified with various levels of psychosexual development, such as the intrusion into the parental couple, separation anxiety, the fear of retaliation and punishment, and the fear of death or ego disintegration (Freud 1926). It is noteworthy that his genesis of anxiety, particularly phobic anxiety, has close connections to the notion of mental space (Freud [1923, S. 26]). He states, 'The ego is first and foremost a bodily ego; it is not merely a surface entity, but is itself the projection of a surface' (Freud 1923, p. 26) and that the first distinctions the primitive ego has to make are those between good and bad, inside and outside, in an attempt to take in the good experiences and to expel the bad ones (Freud 1925).

Other disciples and followers, like Sandor Ferenczi (1922) and Otto Rank (1924), extended Freud's pioneering work. Ernest Jones (1923 [1912], 1923 [1918]) took up Freud's ideas and linked them with the child's curiosity about the contents of the mother's body. Jones also examined the role of symbolism and primitive symbol formation (1916). Helene Deutsch (1929), Edoardo Weiss

(1935), and Bertram Lewin (1933, 1935) added new theories and undertook further exploration with special reference to claustrophobic anxieties. Some of these seminal papers are reprinted in Chapters 1 through 8.

There are many clinicians from different psychoanalytic traditions who have examined the role of mental space and claustrophobic and agoraphobic anxieties from various points of view. In America, Bertram Lewin (1950, 1952, 1953) examined the interiority of the maternal body, intracorporeal anxieties in the nursling situation, dread of being crushed and forced out of this cavity, and the infant's projection of primitive anxieties onto a 'dream screen'. Erik Erikson introduced the term 'claustrum' (Homburger 1937), whose origin Lewin (1950) extended in his concept of the 'oral triad', comprised of the active and passive phantasies of devouring, being devoured, and falling asleep. Lewin's investigations stimulated further work by Jacob Arlow (1960, 1972), Stuart Asch (1966), Robert Fliess (1961, pp. 169–179), Raymond Gehl (1964, 1973), Lucie Jessner (Jessner et al. 1955), and others who applied the concept of mental space to different developmental stages and clinical conditions.

In the British tradition, Ronald Fairbairn (1941, 1952) and Harry Guntrip (1968) linked claustrophobic phenomena with schizoid states and early stages of dependency. Fairbairn viewed agoraphobia and claustrophobia as characteristic fears of abandonment or engulfment when the process of differentiation from the primary object fails. Guntrip (1968, p. 60) described the 'in and out' policy of these patients and the dread they are exposed to when they seek too much closeness in their attempt to evade primitive fears. He observed that schizoid persons are 'extremely liable to fear good and loving relationships more than bad and hostile one' and saw this as 'the reason why they face such exceptional difficulties in personal relationships' (p. 60).

Michael Balint's (1959) description of ocnophilia and philobatia and Donald Winnicott's (1953, 1971) exploration of 'intermediary space', where subjective and objective reality overlap, touch on similar phenomena. Agoraphobic and claustrophobic anxieties relating to early dependency and separation may be counteracted by misrepresenting and erotizing the object relationship. The work of Mervin Glasser (1979, 1986), Masud Khan (1966, 1969), and others explore the attempts at a perverse 'solution' to the claustro-agoraphobic conflict.

In France, André Green (2000) formulated the concept of the 'central phobic position' describing the defences against psychic void and the return of catastrophic anxieties. One of its manifestations in the transference situation is the analyst's feeling that 'the analysand is confused and that he himself is also in danger of becoming confused' (p. 436). In Argentina, Jorge Mom (1956, 1960) examined clinical and technical aspects of the concept of 'distance' in claustrophobia, and Enrique Pichon-Rivière (1971), influenced by Kleinian thought, described a 'relative balance' between the vicious cycle of internal claustrophobic anxiety 'and the agoraphobia anxiety in the outside world' (p. 177). In a similar manner, the German psychoanalyst and philosopher Hermann Lang (1985, 1996) pointed out that the seemingly opposite fears of agoraphobia and claustrophobia are not contradictory but deeply interwoven, relating to the same existential condition.

There are many authors who emphasize the role of an archaic, sadistic super-ego in maintaining primitive claustro-agoraphobic anxieties (Nunberg 1948 [1926], Wurmser 1980, Weiss 2020b). This pathological super-ego can itself serve as a 'claustrum' in which needy and dependent parts of the ego are encaged. Albert Mason (1981) examined this in his paper 'The Suffocating Super-Ego', which is reprinted in Chapter 6 of this book.

Much of this research refers to the theories of Melanie Klein, who had worked with small children during the 1920s in Berlin. She developed the psychoanalytical play technique and, through this methodology, gained immediate access to the phantasy world of her little patients (Frank 2009 [1999]). In these child analyses, Klein discovered that the phantasies of invading or being shut inside the mother's body were quite common and gave rise to archaic fears of punishment and loss (Klein 1975 [1932]). She described a primitive mental organization whose aim was to ensure the survival of the fragile ego by splitting off and projecting those elements that threaten its integrity. At this early stage of development, there is a permanent shift between idealization and persecution, and the borders between self and not-self remain unclear. The individual is mainly concerned with 'part objects', and it is only with the growing integration of loving and hateful impulses that the relationship to a 'whole object', separate from the ego, comes to the fore. With this newly integrated ego, previous fears of ego fragmentation and persecution fade, making room for anxieties of a depressive kind, in particular those of loss and guilt. At this very moment, attempts at 'reparation' converge with the mental process of symbol formation. In 1946, Klein named these two configurations the paranoid-schizoid position and the depressive position and considered them as persisting throughout life.

It is important to note that claustro-agoraphobic anxieties emerge at the border between the paranoid-schizoid and the depressive position. Therefore, they contain both fears of guilt and loss as well as paranoid fears of persecution, fragmentation, and imprisonment. Klein described these anxieties as phantasies of robbing or being robbed, of being attacked inside the mother's body, or as unbearable feelings of loneliness and guilt. Projected parts of the self can remain permanently buried in the object, and claustrophobic anxiety may relate to one's own body if the dangerous objects are localized there (Klein 1975 [1955], 1975 [1963]).

Klein's new model of the human mind deepened and extended Freud's spatial concept of the mental apparatus. In Klein's view, healthy mental development implies a balance between projection and introjection, splitting and integration, which gradually leads to a more realistic picture of the self and the external world. The basic elements of the human mind consist of unconscious phantasies (Isaacs 1948; see Weiss 2017) that continuously evolve over time. Klein (1946) discovered the mechanism of projective identification as a means to expulse and communicate primitive phantasy. Reparation is another important discovery (Klein

1975 [1937]) that assists in the transformation of the archaic super-ego. Analysis of these mental concepts allows for the development of a healthier, more containing structure (Klein 1975 [1958]) essential for psychic development. Finkelstein (Chapter 9) describes the relationship between unconscious phantasy and the concept of reparation in Greek mythology and in Klein's child cases.

One of Klein's disciples, Wilfred R. Bion, extended her clinical findings on infant-mother relating and the role of communicative projective identification (1961, 1962, 1963). Following Klein's (1946, p. 8) suggestion that loving maternal understanding 'contains' and modifies the infant's primitive psychotic anxieties, Bion examined the relationship between container-contained. He postulated a 'semipermeable membrane' mediating and differentiating the internal from the external world. He described the transformation of raw, un-symbolized elements (β-elements) into the precursors of dream thoughts and symbolic thinking (α-elements) through the process of 'containment' (maternal reverie). If this process fails, parts of the self remain locked in the object or are re-introjected in a bizarre form as foreign bodies.

This gives rise to confusion and fears of going mad, which are common in claustro-agoraphobia. Confusional states have been explored by Herbert Rosenfeld (1950, 1965, 1987), whilst Roger Money-Kyrle (1978 [1968]) developed the concept of 'disorientation', which is illustrated in a clinical vignette by Claudia Frank (Chapter 11).

Based on the ideas of Melanie Klein and Wilfred Bion, Donald Meltzer (1966, 1992) developed a version of his own theory of the 'claustrum'. He described the 'geographical confusion' that results when parts of the self are projected and equated with compartments of the mother's body (Chapter 5). As Roger Willoughby (2001a) indicates, Meltzer's ideas refer to Esther Bick's (1953) early thoughts about a tripartite claustral structure that contains the breast, the womb, and the head as its central components (Chapter 4). Referring to Bion's concept of the 'container', Bick later developed her ideas about 'second skin formations' and 'adhesive identification' (Bick 1968, 1986).

Concrete thinking and the failure of proper symbol formation are additional problems that confront claustro-agoraphobic patients. Working with psychotic and borderline patients, Hanna Segal (1957, 1978) examined the process of symbol formation and introduced the term 'symbolic equation'. Henri Rey (1994 [1979], 1994a, 1994b) regarded the persistence of concrete thinking as a central feature in schizoid and claustro-agoraphobic patients. In his seminal paper from 1979 (Chapter 7), Rey both coined the term (which gave the dilemma its name) and introduced the term 'marsupial space' as a space the mother lends the infant to grow and develop, thus facilitating differentiation between the internal and external world. Rey also emphasized the role of reparative processes in overcoming paranoid-schizoid and paranoid anxieties (Rey 1986, 1988).

Like Hanna Segal, Ronald Britton (1989, 1998) emphasized the centrality of the Oedipus complex as the capacity for a third position to foster the development of psychic growth and mental space. It is only when the link between the parental couple is acknowledged that the child can differentiate his own mental space from the space of his mother, thus allowing for true symbolization.

John Steiner's (1993) research on pathological organizations of the personality (Chapter 8) opened the door to a new understanding of claustro-agoraphobic anxieties. He described 'psychic retreats' as interpersonal or mental representations in spatial terms, like an island, dungeon, prison, or cave that the claustro-agoraphobic patient sought as an escape or safe haven. He viewed these complex states of mind as being located at the border between the paranoid-schizoid and depressive positions. He examined the seductive effect these retreats have on the needy parts of the self. Steiner described the different types and levels of anxiety the patient confronts when feeling entrapped in or exiting from this retreat. Steiner's approach had immediate consequences for the understanding of the transference situation and psychoanalytic treatment technique (Steiner 2014).

It is impossible to recognize all the authors who have contributed to the understanding of claustro-agoraphobia, but in his article 'The Dungeon of Thyself: The Claustrum as a Pathological Container', Roger Willoughby (2001b) gives a comprehensive overview of the literature.

For this collection, we have decided to present a selection of classical papers in Chapters 1–8, with contemporary work on claustro-agoraphobia in Chapters 9–12. As the reader will see, there is significant continuity in the evolution of the concept. On the other hand, claustro-agoraphobia is a challenge for the practising analyst, which may contribute to the further development of psychoanalytic technique.

Heinz Weiss (Chapter 10) and Claudia Frank (Chapter 11) present detailed clinical sequences, which give an impression of the difficulties but also of the possible new discoveries one can make in working with these patients. Finally, the Covid-19 pandemic has created a situation in which the limits of time and space are blurred when the analyst works with the patient via the internet or telephone. Kristin White (Chapter 12) explores how these limitations interfere with claustro-agoraphobic anxieties.

As Susan Finkelstein (Chapter 9) reminds us, the claustro-agoraphobic dilemma is not limited to the clinical situation but has a universal meaning in mythology and social anthropology. This may also account for an understanding of war and social conflict when a state or community is suspicious of its neighbours and develops 'a kind of claustrophobia, a feeling of being encircled and shut in' (Roger Money-Kyrle 1978 [1934], p. 133).

References

Arlow, J.A. (1960). Fantasy Systems in Twins. *Psychoanalytic Quarterly, 29*:175–199.
Arlow, J.A. (1972). The Only Child. *Psychoanalytic Quarterly, 41*:507–536.
Asch, S.S. (1966). Claustrophobia and Depression. *Journal of the American Psychoanalytic Association, 14*:711–729.

Balint, M. (1959). *Thrills and Regressions*. London: Hogarth.

Bick, E. (1953). Anxieties Underlying Phobia of Sexual Intercourse in a Woman. *British Journal of Psychotherapy*, *18*(2001):7–21.

Bick, E. (1968). The Experience of Skin in Early Object-Relations. *International Journal of Psychoanalysis*, *49*:484–486.

Bick, E. (1986). Further Considerations on the Function of the Skin in Early Object Relations: Findings from Infant Observation Integrated into Child and Adult Analysis. *British Journal of Psychoanalysis*, *2*:229–299.

Bion, W.R. (1961 [1952]). Group Dynamics. A Re-View. In: Bion, W.R. (1959) (Ed.), *Experiences in Groups and Other Papers*. London: Heinemann.

Bion, W.R. (1962). *Learning from Experience*. London: Heinemann.

Bion, W.R. (1963). *Elements of Psychoanalysis*. London: Heinemann.

Britton, R. (1989). The Missing Link: Parental Sexuality in the Oedipus Complex. In: Steiner, J. (Ed.), *The Oedipus Complex Today: Clinical Implications*. London: Karnac, 83–101.

Britton, R. (1998). *Belief and Imagination: Explorations in Psychoanalysis*. London and New York: Routledge.

Deutsch, H. (1929). The Genesis of Agoraphobia. *International Journal of Psychoanalysis*, *10*:51–69.

Fairbairn, W.R. (1941). A Revised Psychopathology of the Psychoses and Psychoneuroses. *International Journal of Psychoanalysis*, *22*:250–279.

Fairbairn, W.R. (1952). *Psychoanalytic Studies of the Personality*. London: Tavistock Publications Limited.

Ferenczi, S. (1922). Die Brückensymbolik Und Die Don Juan-Legende. *Internationale Zeitschrift Für Psychoanalyse*, *8*:77–78.

Fliess, R. (1961). *Ego and Body Ego. Contributions to Their Psychoanalytic Psychology*. New York: Schulte Publishing Company.

Frank, C. (2009 [1999]). *Melanie Klein in Berlin. Her First Psychoanalyses of Children*. London and New York: Routledge.

Freud, S. (1900). The Interpretation of Dreams. *Standard Edition*, 4–5.

Freud, S. (1916–1917). Introductory Lectures on Psycho-Analysis. *Standard Edition, 15–16*.

Freud, S. (1919). The "Uncanny". *Standard Edition, 17*:217–256.

Freud, S. (1923). The Ego and the Id. *Standard Edition, 19*:12–59.

Freud, S. (1925). Negation. *Standard Edition, 19*:235–239.

Freud, S. (1926). Inhibitions, Symptoms and Anxiety. *Standard Edition, 20*:87–172.

Gehl, R.H. (1964). Depression and Claustrophobia. *International Journal of Psychoanalysis*, *45*:312–323.

Gehl, R.H. (1973). Indecision and Claustrophobia. *International Journal of Psychoanalysis*, *54*:47–59.

Glasser, M. (1979). From the Analysis of a Transvestite. *International Review of Psycho-Analysis*, *6*:163–173.

Glasser, M. (1986). Identification and Its Vicissitudes as Observed in the Perversions. *International Journal of Psychoanalysis*, *67*:9–16.

Green, A. (2000). The Central Phobic Position: A New Formulation of the Free Association Method. *International Journal of Psychoanalysis*, *81*:429–451.

Guntrip, H. (1968). *Schizoid Phenomena, Object-Relations and the Self*. London: Hogarth.

Homburger, E. (1937). Configuration in Play – Clinical Notes. *Psychoanalytic Quarterly*, *6*:139–212.

Isaacs, S. (1948). The Nature and Function of Phantasy. *International Journal of Psychoanalysis, 29*:73–97.

Jessner, L., Lamont, J., Long, R., Rollins, N., Whipple, B., and Prentice, N. (1955). Emotional Impact of Nearness and Separation for the Asthmatic Child and His Mother. *Psychoanalytic Study of the Child, 10*:353–375.

Jones, E. (1916). The Theory of Symbolism. *British Journal of Psychology, 9*:181–239.

Jones, E. (1923 [1912]). A Forgotten Dream: Note on the Oedipus Saving Phantasy. In: Jones, E. (Ed.), *Papers on Psycho-Analysis, 3rd Edition*. London: Bailliere, Tindall and Cox, 255–265.

Jones, E. (1923 [1918]). Anal-Erotic Character Traits. In: Jones, E. (Ed.), *Papers on Psycho-Analysis, 3rd Edition*. London: Bailliere, Tindall and Cox, 680–704.

Khan, M.R. (1966). Role of Phobic and Counterphobic Mechanisms and Separation Anxiety in Schizoid Character Formation. *International Journal of Psychoanalysis, 47*:30.

Khan, M.R. (1969). Role of the "Collated Internal Object" in Perversion-Formations. *International Journal of Psychoanalysis, 50*:555–565.

Klein, M. (1946). Notes on Some Schizoid Mechanisms. In: *The Collected Writings of Melanie Klein, Vol. 3*. London: Hogarth, 1–24.

Klein, M. (1975 [1932]). The Psycho-Analysis of Children. In: *The Collected Writings of Melanie Klein, Vol. 2*. London: Hogarth.

Klein, M. (1975 [1937]). Love, Guilt and Reparation. In: *The Collected Writings of Melanie Klein, Vol. 1*. London: Hogarth, 306–343.

Klein, M. (1975 [1955]). On Identification. In: *The Collected Writings of Melanie Klein, Vol. 3*. London: Hogarth, 141–175.

Klein, M. (1975 [1958]). On the Development of Mental Functioning. In: *The Collected Writings of Melanie Klein, Vol. 3*. London: Hogarth, 236–246.

Klein, M. (1975 [1963]). On the Sense of Loneliness. In: *The Collected Writings of Melanie Klein, Vol. 3*. London: Hogarth, 300–317.

Lang, H. (1985). Zur Struktur Der Angstneurose. In: Bühler, K.-E., and Weiss, H. (Eds), *Kommunikation Und Perspektivität*. Würzburg: Koenigshausen & Neumann, 115–125.

Lang, H. (1996). Zur Pathologie Von Angst Und Angstverarbeitung. In: Lang, H., and Faller, H. (Eds), *Das Phänomen Angst. Pathologie, Genese Und Therapie*. Frankfurt A.M.: Suhrkamp.

Lewin, B.D. (1933). The Body as Phallus. *Psychoanalytic Quarterly, 23*:24–47.

Lewin, B.D. (1935). Claustrophobia. *Psychoanalytic Quarterly, 4*:227–233.

Lewin, B.D. (1950). *The Psychoanalysis of Elevation*. New York: Norton.

Lewin, B.D. (1952). Phobic Symptoms and Dream Interpretation. *Psychoanalytic Quarterly, 21*:295–322.

Lewin, B.D. (1953). Reconsideration of the Dream Screen. *Psychoanalytic Quarterly, 22*:174–199.

Mason, A.A. (1988 [1981]). The Suffocating Superego: Psychotic Break and Claustrophobia. In: Grotstein, J.S. (Ed.), *Do I Dare Disturb the Universe? A Memorial to Wilfred R. Bion*. London: Maresfield, 140–166.

Meltzer, D. (1966). The Relation of Anal Masturbation to Projective Identification. *International Journal of Psychoanalysis, 4*(7):335–342.

Meltzer, D. (1992). The Claustrum. In: *An Investigation of Claustrophobic Phenomena*. Strathtay: Clunie Press.

Mom, J.M. (1956). Algunas Consideraciones Sobre el Concepto de Distancia en las Fobias. *Revista de Psicoanálisis, 13*:430–435.

Mom, J.M. (1960). Aspectos Teóricos y Técnicos en las Fobias y en las Modalidades Fobias. *Revista de Psicoanálisis*, *17*:190–218.

Money-Kyrle, R. (1978 [1934]). A Psychological Analysis of the Causes of War. In: Meltzer, D., and O'Shaughnessy, E. (Eds), *The Collected Papers of Roger Money-Kyrle*. Strathtay: Clunie Press, 131–137.

Money-Kyrle, R. (1978 [1968]). Cognitive Development. In: Meltzer, D., and O'Shaughnessy, E. (Eds), *The Collected Papers of Roger Money-Kyrle*. Strathtay: Clunie Press, 416–433.

Nunberg, H.G. (1948 [1926]). The Sense of Guilt and the Need for Punishment. In: Nunberg, H.G. (Ed.), *Practice and Theory of Psychoanalysis, Vol. 1*. New York: International Universities Press, 89–101.

Rank, O. (1924). The Trauma of Birth in Its Importance for Psychoanalytic Therapy. *Psychoanalytic Review*, *11*:241–245.

Rey, H. (1988). That Which Patients Bring to Analysis. *International Journal of Psychoanalysis*, *69*:457–470.

Rey, H. (1994a). *Universals of Psychoanalysis in the Treatment of Psychotic and Borderline States*. (Hrsg. Magagna, J.). London: Free Association.

Rey, H. (1994b). Basic Schizoid Structures and Space-Time Factors. In: Magagna, J., and Rey, H. (Eds), *Universals of Psychoanalysis in the Treatment of Psychotic and Borderline States*. London: Free Association, 163–175.

Rey, J.H. (1986). Reparation. *Journal of the Melanie Klein Society*, *4*:5–35.

Rey, J.H. (1994 [1979]). Schizoid Phenomena in the Borderline Syndrome. The Schizoid Mode of Being and the Space-Time Continuum. In: Rey, H. (Ed.), *Universals of Psychoanalysis in the Treatment of Psychotic and Borderline States* (Ed. Magagna, J.). London: Free Association, 8–30.

Rivière, E.P. (1971). The Link and the Theory of the Three Ds (Depositant, Depositary, and Deposited): Role and Status. *International Journal of Psychoanalysis*, *98*(2017):177–186.

Rosenfeld, H.A. (1950). Note on the Psychopathology of Confusional States in Chronic Schizophrenias. *International Journal of Psychoanalysis*, *31*:132–137.

Rosenfeld, H.A. (1965). Psychotic States. In: *A Psychoanalytical Approach*. London: Hogarth.

Rosenfeld, H.A. (1987). *Impasse and Interpretation: Therapeutic and Anti-Therapeutic Factors in the Psychoanalytic Treatment of Psychotic, Borderline, and Neurotic Patients*. London: Tavistock Publications.

Segal, H. (1957). Notes on Symbol Formation. *International Journal of Psychoanalysis*, *38*:391–397.

Segal, H. (1978). On Symbolism. *International Journal of Psychoanalysis*, *59*:315–319.

Steiner, J. (1993). *Psychic Retreats: Pathological Organizations in Psychotic, Neurotic and Borderline Patients*. London and New York: Routledge.

Steiner, J. (2014 [2011]). Das Betäubende Gefühl Von Wirklichkeit. In: Steiner, J., and Seelische Rückzugsorte Verlassen (Eds), *Therapeutische Schritte Zur Aufgabe Der Borderline-Position* (Hrsg. Weiß, H., and Frank, C.). Stuttgart: Klett-Cotta, 77–96.

Weiss, E. (1935). Agoraphobia and Its Relation to Hysterical Attacks and to Traumas. *International Journal of Psychoanalysis*, *16*:59–83.

Weiss, H. (2017). Unconscious Phantasy as a Structural Principle and Organizer of Mental Life: The Evolution of a Concept from Freud to Klein and Some of Her Successors. *International Journal of Psychoanalysis*, *98*:799–819.

Weiss, H. (2020a [2009]). *Trauma, Guilt and Reparation. The Path from Impasse to Development*. London and New York: Routledge; Stuttgart: Klett-Cotta.

Weiss, H. (2020b). A Brief History of the Super-Ego with an Introduction to Three Papers. *International Journal of Psychoanalysis*, *101*:724–734.

Willoughby, R. (2001a). The Petrified Self: Esther Bick and Her Membership Paper. *British Journal of Psychotherapy*, *18*:3–6.

Willoughby, R. (2001b). "The Dungeon of Thyself": The Claustrum as Pathological Container. *International Journal of Psychoanalysis*, *82*:917–931.

Winnicott, D.W. (1953). Transitional Objects and Transitional Phenomena – A Study of the First Not-Me Possession. *International Journal of Psychoanalysis*, *34*:89–97.

Winnicott, D.W. (1971). *Playing and Reality*. London: Tavistock.

Wurmser, L. (1980). Phobic Core in the Addictions and the Paranoid Process. *International Journal of Psychoanalysis*, *62*:311–335.

Chapter 1

The Genesis of Agoraphobia[1]

Helene Deutsch

SUMMARY

Agoraphobia is the genuine dread of death to oneself or one's love object. Deutsch places agoraphobia in an intermediate position between obsessional neurosis and conversion hysteria. She emphasizes the early infantile relation to the primary love object and the fear of losing it. In her case studies of female agoraphobic patients, Deutsch discusses the primitive form of identification with a maternal object and its sadomasochistic defences and wishes to protect and kill the object or one's own ego. Deutsch opines that the agoraphobe's wish to be accompanied by a 'particular' companion unconsciously represents a regression from genitality to oral and anal sadistic defences to control one's violent obsessional sadistic and castrative impulses toward the loved object. Through the process of identification and reversal, the agoraphobe feels panic when in the street without a companion to protect against sexual, oedipal, and exhibitionist desire. The 'protection' of the 'special companion' is a lightly veiled disguise for regression from the Oedipus to earlier merged states with the mother and the threat of separation by its disturber, the father. Published in 1929, this article suggests Deutsch may have had knowledge of Klein's 1928 findings of the early maternal Oedipus complex. In agoraphobia, fear of intercourse symbolizes the union between the parents or retribution for oedipal (positive and negative) longings. Deutsch describes both the aggressive impulse to harm the mother and its anti-cathexis in the reaction formation of over-anxious tenderness. She considers both the emotional and spatial presence and absence of the object as releasing regressive dependent hostile oedipal and pre-oedipal anal impulses.

She stresses the process of mutual scrutinizing in suspicious 'watchfulness'. In this interchange, the super-ego becomes the 'protector under protection'.

Deutsch stresses working with the positive and negative transference in order to work through the multiple layers of identification with the object. One can see the effect of her psychoanalytic thinking about female sexuality, parturition, frigidity, and intercourse in Edoardo Weiss (Chapter 3), Esther Bick (Chapter 4), and Mason's (Chapter 6) concept of the 'suffocating super-ego' and the perverse omnipotent, omniscient, and omnipresent control of 'watching' the other.

DOI: 10.4324/9781003200284-1

Deutsch's later studies of emotional disturbance (1942) and the 'as if' personality can be intuited in this 1929 paper, as she theorizes the agoraphobic condition as an 'intermediate position' (p. 51). One can see the effect of her thinking on all future analysts, including Henri Rey's concepts of spatial and ego disturbances in borderline patients (Chapter 7).

TEXT

The observations which I have recorded in this paper have reference to a very definite type of illness, the symptoms of which may be described as follows: There are certain people who, when left to themselves in the street, experience the most intense anxiety. All the different symptoms of anxiety ensue: palpitation, trembling and, above all, the feeling that they are on the point of collapsing, that their end is near and they are helpless to avert it. Their anxiety is a genuine dread of death, and the content of their phobia, if put into words, is this: 'I shall suddenly die'. In this situation the terrifying thought grips them that they are on the verge of a fainting fit, a heart-attack, a stroke or some other catastrophe. Often the anxiety centres in the idea that they will be run over, will meet with a railway or a motor accident, and so forth. It is characteristic of this condition that it either totally disappears or becomes far less acute if the patient has somebody with him. Sometimes he derives a sense of security from being within sight of his home. As a rule, the person with him must fulfil certain conditions to be of any use. There must be an affectionate relation between the two of them. Many people suffering from agoraphobia insist on being accompanied by a particular person. Others seem to be less hard to satisfy and will be contented with anyone whom they can associate with the prospect of 'speedy help'. Rich patients want to know that their physician, together with the salvation of his hypodermic syringe, is near at hand.

Since there appeared to be nothing remarkable in such patients' choice of a companion, we have hitherto been satisfied with their assertion that the possibility of rescue was the important point, and we paid no further attention to this 'subordinate figure'. In this paper I propose to discuss three cases which I knew intimately and in which certain circumstances impelled me to examine more closely into the significance of the 'companion'. I thus made some discoveries (which I think are important) about the nature of agoraphobia. I will not anticipate my conclusions, but will just say a little more about the general characteristics of such patients.

Apart from the state of anxiety, which arises only when they are in the street, these patients are for all practical purposes normal. It is interesting to note that the disposition of some of them is more like that of the obsessional neurotic, while that of others is markedly hysterical. Cases with pronounced obsessional symptoms, existing side by side with those typical of agoraphobia (like the case described by Alexander[2]), are very common, and it is equally common to find a combination of agoraphobia with conversion-symptoms and hysterical attacks.

These observations suggest that agoraphobia occupies an intermediate position between these two forms of illness.

I will now examine and compare certain cases from the point of view of the affinity of agoraphobia to obsessional neurosis on the one hand and hysteria on the other.

The first case is that of a girl of twenty, an only child. The father, who obviously took no interest in family life, had married a very wealthy woman and was in the position of a guest in his own house. The mother, who was highly neurotic, had from the outset concentrated all her unsatisfied libido on the child. The early infantile relation which existed between mother and child before the Oedipus complex made its appearance had been so successfully preserved that, at the time of treatment, the patient still slept with her mother and, when going to sleep, would suck at her mother's breast or finger. The analysis was mainly occupied with this relation between the two and aimed at resolving the morbid mother-fixation by producing a mother-transference. During the whole time of treatment, the father stood for one thing only: an extremely unwelcome disturber of the peace, who at times threatened to come between the patient and her mother. In any case the Oedipus complex had terminated in a reinforcement of the mother-fixation.

In the anamnesis the mother said that the patient could never bear her to be away and that really, ever since her daughter's birth, she had been a slave to her. But it was not until the child reached puberty that the morbid symptoms appeared. She began to display intense anxiety if her mother left the house, the content of the anxiety being that something might happen to her mother, 'she might, for instance, be run over'. The daughter was always waiting for her at the window with a tense expression and heaved a sigh of joy and relief when she saw her safe and sound. To those versed in analytic work it is clear that this exaggeratedly affectionate anxiety was of the nature of an over-compensation and must be regarded as a hysterical reaction-formation. The sensations of anxiety and the ideas about her mother dying in the street remind us of agoraphobia, but the roles are divided; the anxiety is experienced by the subject, while it is the object who is in danger of death.[3]

Thus our patient's first neurotic symptom had been a hysterical one. Her anxiety doubtless had reference to the threatened loss of the love-object, her ambivalent feelings towards that object already showing plainly in the content of her anxiety: something frightful was happening to her mother. This relation to her mother was an extension of the early infantile relation, and the genital repression of puberty was directed above all against homosexual impulses.

After the first, hysterical phase of her neurosis there followed, as we shall see, a transformation of her symptoms, which took on the colour of obsessional neurosis. In the analysis one could clearly trace the regressive revival of sadistic-anal tendencies after the successful repression of the genital ones. But, before this happened, yet another symptom-formation of the hysterical type could be recognized. The patient became unable to go out herself without her mother, the reason she gave being that, while she was out, something 'dreadful' might happen to her mother (through her father, as we discovered in the analysis). The new symptom differed from the first only in the reversal of the locations: the patient now was in the street and the mother at home. The content was the same: once more this anxiety concerning the mother consisted of dread of a loss. That is to say, she feared lest in her absence the mother might bestow her love on the father. The hate-tendencies against the mother represented, on the one hand, a reaction to disappointment, and, on the other, were certainly part of the normal Oedipus complex, though in this patient it was buried deep beneath the impulses belonging to the inverted form of the complex.

This hysterical symptom, in its changed form, was, moreover, closely related to agoraphobia. The patient could not go out alone, because of her anxiety lest, while she was out, some mischance might happen to her mother. The close affinity between the two lies in the fact that this patient too was overtaken with anxiety if her 'companion' (her mother) was not with her. Only the content is different: it was not she herself who was threatened with some fearful disaster, but the person whom she longed to have with her and who had stayed at home.

So far the patient's symptoms showed a certain likeness to the clinical picture of agoraphobia. In the sequel a constellation arose which, on the one hand, increased this similarity, but, on the other hand, plainly contained considerable differences. The patient had already reached the stage of not being able to go out without her mother; the next stage differed in that, even when they were together, she was tormented with the most intense anxiety about her mother, whom she held encircled convulsively by her arm, always concerned lest some accident should happen to her. Finally, the obsessional impulse which had so far been held in check broke out. She was seized with anxiety lest *she herself* should push her mother in front of a tram or a motor. This obsessive fear was combined with the obsessive impulse actually to do so.

In this case we can observe the transformation of one form of neurosis into another, the content of both being the aggressive impulse, which is repressed in the first form, only an anti-cathexis manifesting itself in the reaction-formation of over-anxious tenderness. Here the anxiety has its origin in two commingling tendencies. The one is a continuation of the early infantile relation to the love-object and a response to the danger of losing it. The other is a danger-signal, indicating the presence of the sadistic impulse and bringing about a further over-compensation by tenderness. The presence of the object is the necessary condition of the patient's relief from anxiety. The neurotic symptom, so long as it was hysterical, consisted simply in this. We assume that in the further course of the neurosis a regression to the anal-sadistic phase occurred, which, we believe, explains the break-through of the impulse.

I will now pass on to the cases of agoraphobia proper. The first was handed over to me some years ago by a colleague who was leaving Vienna. The patient was a young girl with symptoms of typical agoraphobia. Whenever she went out without her parents she was seized with the most acute anxiety (of the kind that I have already described). Either her father or her mother had to accompany her.

According to her own statement her first anxiety-attack in the street occurred when she saw a man fall down in an epileptic fit. From that time on she was unable to recover from the shock of this sight, especially as she was constantly hearing of cases of sudden death and seemed to be peculiarly unlucky in perpetually meeting ambulances or funerals and being reminded anew, by these 'experiences', of the possibility of her own death. It is indeed remarkable how often persons suffering from agoraphobia are startled by such apparently fortuitous incidents which have a traumatic effect on them. It really is that their attention is turned in a particular direction, and thus they are always ready to receive these impressions, while other people do not notice them – the patients themselves may thus have the idea that they are pursued by a peculiar ill-luck. As regards the particular patient of whom I am speaking, I must mention that at about the time that she fell ill, that is, something like a year before the treatment, she began an erotic relation with a young man, which the bourgeois morality of her parents sanctioned as long as it remained a 'platonic friendship'.

During the patient's treatment by her first analyst there was a considerable improvement in her condition. Obviously this was a success due to the transference, and the meaning of it became clear as the analysis proceeded. The sympathetic and kindly treatment, which during the first part of her analysis acted as a substitute-gratification for her libidinal relation with her father, had resulted in her being able to come to analysis by herself and to go about within a considerable radius of the analyst's house without anxiety. The vivid, conscious phantasy about the analyst acted as a wish-fulfilment and served as a protection against anxiety and a substitute for a companion. Soon after Dr. X. went away, a fresh accession of anxiety occurred, this time with an unexpected content – namely, that something might happen to him on his journey: he might, for instance, have a heart-attack. For a time, the preoccupation with his personal safety submerged the thought of her own. At this point I might already indicate the analogy with the first phase of the case I described before. But in the second patient this phase of the illness was a passing one and was soon succeeded by the original clinical picture: anxiety about herself. In the first patient, on the other hand, the illness developed into an obsessional neurosis. This, as I said before, was owing to a regression to the pregenital phase. But in the case of the girl suffering from agoraphobia what was the determining factor in the clinical picture?

Let me point out, first of all, that the analyst's departure was felt by the patient as a disappointment in love and produced a sadistic reaction, which was, however, repudiated and converted into anxious concern for him. This apprehensiveness corresponded to the hysterical reaction-formation which I have already mentioned. The fact that the content of the anxiety was in both instances the same – first, about herself and then about the love-object who frustrated her libidinal desires – leads us to suppose that there must be some element which bridged the gulf between the two ideas connected with the anxiety.

The patient's analysis grouped itself round two traumatic experiences. The first occurred in the very middle of her childhood, while the second dominated her adolescence. The infantile experience was the actual overhearing of intercourse between her parents, when she imagined that her father was strangling and torturing her mother. The incident at puberty was a severe seizure which her father had after a bath. He collapsed as though dead and had to go to a sanatorium for a considerable time. All the patient's phantasies at the time of puberty were the revival of the situation when, as a child, she listened to her parents. They were of a feminine, masochistic tone and contained, besides the normal ideas of the man's overpowering the woman and degrading her to the status of a prostitute, other specially blood-thirsty features: for instance, that a red-hot iron bar was thrust into her genital, that she gave birth to a child and in doing so burst into pieces.

In all these masochistic phantasies which the patient had woven round the experience of overhearing parental coitus she had identified herself with her mother. The Oedipus complex terminated in the fixation of this identification and of the desire associated with it to get rid of the mother. In this patient the desire took an especially aggressive form. The experience during puberty (her father's sudden illness) which befell her at the time when the conflicts of puberty had set in, had revived the memory of the early infantile experience and mobilized again the former (hitherto repressed) reactions to that episode, in so far as they affected her attitude to her father. Her wish might be formulated thus: 'If you do not love me as you did my mother, then you shall die'. Her father's loss of consciousness and the convulsions with which he was seized were precisely the connecting link of association with the first, infantile scene. The *repudiated* death-wish against the father corresponded to the regressive revival of the infantile desire to castrate him.

The neurosis broke out after she had in real life been approached sexually by her lover. The object of the symptom was that her parents should protect her 'in the street' (i.e. outside the house) from a danger which there was now actual reason to apprehend. But this did not exhaust their duty as companions. As soon as the patient was placed in a situation of temptation (i.e. outside the shelter of her parents' house), mobilization occurred of the instinctual impulses which at other times she kept firmly in a state of repression.

As we have seen, these impulses were predominantly masochistic in character. The danger to the ego lay not only in the particular impulse which she repudiated, but in the destructive tendencies of the instinct. We have seen that the Oedipus constellation, which had been retained by fixation and to which the patient regressed, had for its basis a feminine-masochistic identification with the mother. The result of this was that even the patient's aggressive tendencies, whose real object was the mother, were turned against her own ego, transformed as it was by identification. In addition, the aggressive impulses directed against herself received reinforcement from her hostility to her father.

There was particularly clear evidence of this last fact in the girl's transference-relation to Dr. X. The analyst's sympathetic response to her difficulties and her hope and expectation of winning his love had modified the aggressive tendencies and set her free from anxiety. When frustration occurred, all her sadistic, revengeful feelings were roused up again and the anxiety acquired a content nearer to its source. The kind of death to which she condemned the analyst corresponded perfectly to the impression made on the patient by her father's seizure and further to what she feared for herself in her phobia.

The whole, adequately repressed, material became mobilized only under certain conditions. When she was separated from her parents the street (which to her mind was a 'situation of temptation' partly in reality and partly symbolically) constituted the dangerous condition. We can now understand why the anxiety which had reference to dangers within herself was allayed when she had her parents with her. The ostensible protection from the external dangers of the street was simply a gross rationalization – a displacement to the outside world.

Her identification with her mother, which was determined by the mode of her libidinal development, contained two sources of danger: that of loss of the love-object and that of death to her own ego through a reversed direction of her aggressive tendencies. Her mother's actual presence seemed to diminish both dangers: the first by virtue of the reassurance obtained from the loving protection she bestowed, and from the certainty of her still existing as a love-object in the outside world, and the second (that of the girl's own death) in that the patient, while herself sheltered by her mother, was enabled in her turn to protect the latter, and therefore her own 'ego' also. At the conclusion of this paper, I will come back to the considerations that I have thus briefly sketched.

Case III. The patient whose case I shall now describe was a woman of about forty, of the lower middle class, the mother of three children. Hitherto she had been practically well and normal. Her elder daughter, a girl of seventeen, who had been brought up by her mother on lines of strict bourgeois morality, was beginning to be interested in men and love and all the things which are of the greatest importance at her age. This disquieted the mother, who, although she seemed to permit her daughter these interests, was continually spying on her and weaving the web of her own curiosity around the girl's innocent love-life. Finally, she learnt from her daughter's diary, which she discovered 'accidentally', that the girl was just forming a relation with a man for whom the patient herself cherished a certain interest. Thereupon her neurosis set in. To me it was extraordinarily interesting to note how the whole conscious and unconscious phantasy-life of this woman, who was approaching the climacteric, was dominated by the revived emotions of puberty. In typical fashion the daughter assumed in the patient's phantasy-life the position which the patient's mother had once occupied. There arose in this woman, who was almost elderly, the characteristic phantasies of puberty (defloration, rape and prostitution), phantasies, that is, of all those dangers which she, as an anxious mother, should properly have dreaded for her daughter. These impulses of the patient's illicit desires (which she repudiated) constituted an identification between herself and her daughter. At the same time the latter became her hated rival, against whom she directed the whole revenge-reaction, which originally had reference to her own mother and had been suppressed. In imagination (almost conscious) she saw in her daughter, as she had once seen in her mother, an obstacle in the path of her own happiness. She used to tell me that she had been brought up by her mother quite differently from 'modern' girls. She was not allowed to go out without a companion, and a strict watch was kept upon any love-affairs. This same situation of being watched was what she repeated in her agoraphobia. It was impossible for her, tortured as she was by the dread of death, to go out alone. The only person she would have taken as a companion was this daughter, but as actual circumstances prevented the patient's insisting on this condition, the result was that she generally had to give up going out.

Here we can perceive with remarkable clearness how the different roles are allotted. The daughter is to be on the watch and see that the mother does not succumb to her instinctual impulses, the very ones which constitute the basis of identification between the two. In our patient there are not only the dangers arising out of the promptings of instinct, but also the aggressive wish to get rid of the rival; owing to the identification which has been established, the fury of this desire is turned upon the ego. At the same time the mother is keeping a watch on her daughter, in whose situation the element of danger lies not merely in her awakening sexuality (which it is the mother's duty to protect), but also in that mother's unconscious aggressive impulses. Thus the daughter has assumed also the role of the super-ego, the vigilant faculty, the guardian who forbids and menaces – the role which was formerly filled by the patient's mother. We see here a process analogous to that in the case described earlier in this paper. The companion becomes the 'protector under protection'. The fact that the object of the identification, against whom the aggressive tendency is directed, is set up in the outside world and that its guardianship takes a loving and not a menacing form, enables the patient to lose her dread of death. The process of identification on the one hand and, on the other, the threat of death to the subject's own ego are transitory manifestations associated with the situation of temptation arising when the patient is out-of-doors. It is noteworthy that her feelings of anxiety were at first associated only with a certain part of her way from home – a path along by a fence behind which she often saw men urinating. My reason for emphasizing this is that I have received the impression that exhibitionistic tendencies play an important (though subordinate) part in the determination of street-perils. I will come back to this point in telling you the next case-history.

Case IV. This was the case of a woman, aged twenty-seven, who had been married for three years. She was the second of three children and had a brother two years older than herself, in relation to whom a marked penis-envy had developed. Of her sister, two years younger than herself, she was acutely envious on the oral level. Both these hate-relations had a very crippling effect on her life. When she was four and a half, her brother died after an operation on the cæcum. His death caused the fixation in her mind of a most crushing sense of guilt, the more so as other critical events in her childhood came to be associated with him. Chief amongst these was a great disappointment inflicted on her by her mother. She had thought that, when her brother died, she would win her mother for herself, but, instead, she lost her. For the mother, utterly overwhelmed with grief, withdrew from her family and lived by herself in an attic room. This separation placed the little daughter in a situation which she had doubtless wished for, but which was full of danger. The little girl now slept in her father's bed and was able to translate into reality quite a considerable part of her Oedipus phantasies. After a year the mother tried to resume family life, whereupon she found already in her little daughter neurotic reactions to these occurrences. During the latency-period further neurotic difficulties arose: a dread of thunder and of earthquakes and all kinds of slight conversion-symptoms, which analysis showed to be phantasies of pregnancy. Even before puberty the child had heard of women who walk the streets at night and do something 'dreadful', and she could not be induced to leave the house in the evening. Her imaginings about these women underwent condensation with the phantasy which depreciates the mother; thus the mother was degraded to the level of a prostitute.

Two recollections from the latency-period played a great part in her analysis. The one was about an anxiety-attack in the street on a certain occasion when her mother had told her to go and apologize to a lady from whose garden she had stolen some fruit. She obeyed with fury in her heart, but she failed to carry out her mother's injunction because on the way she was seized with palpitation and trembling. She realized herself that it was a question of suppressed rage against both women.

The other recollection was associated with a story called 'The Lighthouse-keeper'. There was a certain lighthouse of which the keeper was a woman. Her duty was to give warning signals to the ships at sea. She lived in the lighthouse alone with her little daughter. One day the little girl found her mother up in the tower, lying on the ground dead. The woman had died suddenly of a heart attack in the midst of carrying out her important duties. The courageous child, with great presence of mind, took upon herself her mother's work and heroically saved the ships which were in peril.

After reading this story the patient was seized with the most acute anxiety whenever her mother went out, and would stand at the window or the gate until her mother came back. We note here the same condition as in the case of the first patient (the one with the obsessional neurosis), but the sequel was different. In an extremely characteristic way, the patient would say of her phobia: 'I do not know whether the anxiety was for myself or my mother'. The content of the story shows clearly what was the content of this anxiety. The little girl in the book took her mother's place. The death of the mother was the condition of an unconscious wish-fulfilment in the patient herself. At the same time the role which she tried to enact as a substitute for her mother was associated with the same depreciation and degradation of her own person as she originally applied to her mother. The fulfilment of these wishes would make the patient herself a prostitute, as in her phantasy she made her mother. We recall the infantile situation which was undoubtedly the traumatic basis of her neurosis. Although this situation appears to be a quite individual experience, it not only gives its cast to the subsequent neurosis of this particular patient, but also affords a rough outline of my conception of agoraphobia. As a little girl the patient was abandoned by her mother, on whom she was very dependent. This constituted a trauma – the loss of the love-object. The mother left her place beside the father to the child, who was thus exposed by her to the danger of fulfilment of her unconscious wishes which culminated in identification with the mother.

When the mother came back from her voluntary exile the little girl's mind was already ripe for rivalry: she could maintain her place under one condition only, namely, if her mother died, like the light-house-keeper. (The very relation between the places where the two women lived formed an analogy: the attic was equivalent to the tower.) In later life, when situations arose which contained the potential gratification of the patient's repressed libidinal tendencies (which in her, as in the other cases, were of a masochistic nature), she summoned her mother from exile. The intention was twofold: first, that she might prevent the fulfilment of these wishes and, secondly, lest the death-wish, conceived in the past against the mother, whether in her role of protectress or as the person interfering with the child's gratification, should be fulfilled with the patient herself as the victim. The anxiety-signal of her agoraphobia was nothing else but her past summons to her mother.

Let us now return to the history of the case. While still at school she entered into a sentimental love-relation with a boy schoolfellow. At the age of eighteen she made the acquaintance of her future husband, who made a strong sexual impression on her and began to woo her. This led to a conflict. The home atmosphere of her childhood was prodigiously ascetic and bigoted. After the death of her son the mother had visibly adopted a neurotic type of asceticism. Whilst practising self-denial herself, she became excessively strict in questions of morality, and everything to do with sex was placed under the severest ban. A conflict now arose in the patient's mind when her passionless relation to her friend was interrupted by her future husband. For the friendship she already had her mother's permission, which amounted to a command that one was bound to remain faithful to one's first, 'ideal' love. The patient could not make up her mind one way or the other. Clearly the relation to her future husband was prohibited, even on external grounds, since he, in contrast to her devout mother, was an atheist. The conflict assumed a neurotic character and the patient tried to find a way out. She had already conceived the idea that, if she broke with her friend, it would kill him. That is to say, she was already endeavouring to get the disturber of her wishes 'out of the way like her brother'. As a prophylactic measure for relieving herself of the sense of guilt she underwent the same operation as that to which her brother had succumbed. This had the mental effect of enabling her to come to a decision: she broke with her friend and became happily engaged to the other man. Thereupon the agoraphobia broke out. One Sunday, when she was going to see a motherly friend (the patient lived a long way from her own home) to tell her of her deliverance from conflict, she was troubled on the way by the idea: 'What will she think of my behaviour?' Deep in thought, she came into a rather quiet street and was suddenly seized with a feeling of dread: 'I am going to collapse utterly'. Her friend had to be fetched, and only under her protection could the patient go the rest of the way.

Now, what had happened? Her break with her schoolfellow had caused her sense of guilt to weigh very heavily upon her and had revived the memory of her brother's death. By breaking off the friendship she was enabling herself to gratify her sexual desires, as she had done when she slept with her father. Hence all these desires took on an infantile character and came under a severe prohibition. As in the early episode, her mother would cease to love her and would abandon her to sexual danger. As then, so now, the death-wish against the mother awoke in her mind. As in the first, infantile phase of her neurosis, to which I have alluded, she waited in suspense for her mother, so now she could not go a step further without being protected and delivered by her from the sense of blood-guiltiness. This was why the friend – a mother-imago – had to accompany her.

The neurosis settled down into a typical agoraphobia. Acting on medical advice, she married the man she loved, but her state became, if anything, worse. Her only gain was that her husband became to her the companion whom she tormented with her symptoms and chained to her side. Coitus brought on acute anxiety-attacks and vaginismus.

In her analysis with me she soon developed a wonderful 'transference-neurosis', which, through the many details of her relation to myself, gave me considerable insight into the original neurosis.

The first phase was dominated by a 'negative transference' refusal to be cured with me as analyst and distrust of my tolerance. How (she asked) could I be a proper analyst when I forbade my own daughter (as the patient phantasied) everything to do with sex? She interpreted my every gesture as a prohibition and oscillated between flat refusal and slavish obedience. She always entirely confirmed my interpretations, but I noticed that often (for instance, before she told some dream which was in striking agreement with what I had said) she began to laugh convulsively and frequently a quarter of an hour would pass before she could stop. It was clear that, while ostensibly accepting me, she was really distrustful and was mocking me.

If I gave her any piece of advice, e.g. that she should be examined by a gynæcologist, she fell into a state of obsessional indecision: she was forced to obey and yet she could not bring herself to go. One day I did actually ask her to come to me on foot and not, as she usually did, by motor. Nevertheless on the way she took a taxi, but on this occasion, contrary to her custom, she was seized in the taxi also with acute anxiety, the dread being that she would be punished with death because she had transgressed my order. On the steps she was overcome by the feeling that something had happened to *me*. For the first time she had an anxiety-attack during analysis. It gradually passed into a typical tonic-clonic hysterical attack and she fell on the floor. When the attack ended, she knelt before me and said: 'Forgive me'. I asked her what there was for me to forgive and she replied: 'My temper'. Thus, it was obvious that the attack was a vent for her rage.

On this day she went away perfectly free from anxiety for the first time in seven years; it is to be noted that she had never before had a hysterical fit. The next few days passed almost without anxiety and the patient constructed a 'ceremonial' about myself, in order to remain free. For instance, when walking in the street she would keep close to women in whom her imagination could see me. But she avoided any woman who looked 'feeble', in case this woman should 'collapse'. Or the patient would remain for hours in the neighbourhood of my house and would experience no anxiety. A visiting-card of mine was used by her as a protective talisman, as a bit of myself. The head of the pension which I had recommended to her received from her a certain amount of transference-feeling. The patient would go out with her, but with a sense of oppression and anxiety lest this lady should collapse in the street. The way to my house was divided into two halves. The first was beset with anxiety and in the middle there was a gap which greatly increased this emotion; from that point on there was a safe zone.

As the positive transference grew, her anxiety increased lest I should inevitably turn her out if I discovered everything. Next, she produced phantasies in which *I* did all the things which were forbidden her. For instance, she phantasied that I had secret relations with men, that I had love-affairs with my male patients and stripped myself in their presence, and one day she confessed under great resistance that she had an idea that I masturbated during the analytic hour. All these accusations corresponded to her own wish-phantasies and established an identity between the two of us by way of the idea of guilt in common. My other side, too, with its hypermorality and its prohibitions, corresponded to the patient's own ascetic ego-ideal. This dissociation in my personality was identical with that which she had formerly contrived in her thoughts about her mother and made the basis of her identification with her. On the one hand were all the forbidden, sexual tendencies and, on the other, the severe, menacing super-ego. The furious death-wish against me was (as analysis showed) part of the revolt against the mother and was converted into a threat of death to her own ego, which she identified with the mother.

In the following dream we have an especially clear illustration of this identification of her mother with myself:

> She was lying on a hard bedstead, with her feet close to a fire-place which was a combination of a stove and a gas-fire. The bedstead was made out of two chairs which were pushed apart so that part of her back was in the air. A burning candle stood on the ground below this part of her back, which she had to keep on arching in order not to be burnt. She had palpitation and a sense of anxiety.

The patient's associations to this dream led to the situation of danger to which her mother had exposed her when, after the little son's death, she gave up sleeping on the same floor as the father and daughter. The father (who was evidently the victim of an obsessional neurosis) used always to look under the bed at night with a lighted candle. The motions which the patient made in the dream corresponded to the typical *arc de cercle*, reproduced in her hysterical attack during the analytic hour. The fire-place at her feet was a condensation of a stove in the room where

I treated her and a kitchen-grate at home. At her mother's wish she was obliged to cook the breakfast on this kitchen-stove and, while doing so, she had a great dread of mice which used to creep out of holes under the grate.

In this dream the patient was trying to shift on to her mother's shoulders the blame for her own onanism and her phantasies relating to her father. Her mother had in fact brought her into these situations, but I was repeating the offence by making her phantasies conscious.

In another dream

> she was lying in bed with her mother and perceived that the latter was mas-
> turbating. The patient took her mother's hand away from the genitals and
> woke with feelings of anxiety.

Here we see clearly the identification between the dreamer and her mother on the one hand and, on the other, between myself and the mother (by way of the masturbation-phantasy, which, as I have mentioned, the patient had about me).

As her relation with me gradually lost the strain of anxiety, she ventured to reveal to me more and more her sexual phantasies. These were throughout on the genital level, feminine and markedly masochistic in character and the birth-phantasy, both in its active and passive forms, was of central significance in her agoraphobia. Hysterical attacks which developed during the analytic hour gave access to the hidden content of her agoraphobia.

Such attacks would take place, for example, when she was relating anxiety-dreams, or the attacks themselves would be of a dream-like nature and, when they passed, the patient would be able to tell me the content of the phantasy which had accompanied them. These dreams and phantasies were representations of parturition. For instance, she dreamt that

> she was in a dark cellar. She was pursued by some woman and experienced
> awful anxiety because she could not escape from the cellar. Suddenly she saw
> that blood was flowing from a 'hole in her head'. An ambulance was standing
> outside; she was placed in it and felt that she was saved.

Her associations made it plain that the dream represented parturition. In another dream, the narrating of which brought on an attack,

> she was standing by a window and was surprised to find that she felt anxiety
> lest she should fall through it. She threw a little doll through the window in
> the street, whereupon she felt that she was at the point of death. This feeling
> was warded off by vigorous jerks of her whole body.

What was especially interesting in this case was its gradual conversion into hysteria, manifested in recurring attacks. As her relation to me improved and the destructive function of the now more submissive super-ego became more restricted, the anxiety diminished. Every time some repressed content was aroused by the analysis, hysterical attacks occurred, but, characteristically, *only* during the analytic hour. These attacks represented situations of a distinctly genital character (onanism, coitus, birth, parturition). The patient said that she could allow herself to have attacks while she was with me because, even though it was like dying, she had no need to fear when I was there. When she was out in the street the anxiety seemed necessary as a protection from the fulfilment of unconscious tendencies. I think we may accept her explanation. So long as the aggressive tendencies of her super-ego were holding over her the threat of death, the wish-impulses had to be prohibited. But when the tension between ego and super-ego (i.e. in the analytic situation, between her and myself) grew less, the permissive forces could come into play and she could allow herself to represent the repressed instinctual wishes in symbolic form in her attacks. I think that the modification of her aggressive tendencies by analysis had this result: the super-ego became less severe, the genital impulses could fulfil themselves and motor discharge in the hysterical attacks took the place of the inhibiting anxiety.

In this case we see the conversion of one form of neurosis into another, just as in the case I described first anxiety-hysteria was metamorphosed into obsessional impulses. At first, the inner danger of the sadistic tendencies was held in check by the exaggeratedly tender anxiety about the imperilled love-object. When the repressed ideational content broke through, the aggressive tendencies became conscious and could be combated by external measures. In Alexander's opinion[4] the murderous impulses break through the repression when the ego, in consequence of punishment inflicted on it by the super-ego, has lost its power of resistance to the id, but, on the other hand, when by what it has suffered it has satisfied the claims of the super-ego (in the guise of conscience) and can afford to admit the repressed impulses to consciousness. In the case of the patient with obsessive impulses, discussed earlier in this paper, it looks as though the breaking-through into consciousness depended on yet another condition. So long as the mechanism by which the forbidden impulses were kept in the unconscious was applied, in a manner typical of hysteria, to the sense of guilt as well, the hostile tendency could remain concealed under the guise of anxious concern for the object threatened with danger.

When the destructive tendencies are reinforced by regression, the hard-pressed ego tries to find a rational justification for its feelings of guilt which are pressing towards consciousness. Just as the 'criminal from sense of guilt' tries to manufacture a real ground for it in the external world in order to rationalize his guilt, so the hard-pressed ego seeks to find in its own internal world a rationalization for its sense of guilt. In its search for the motive of this guilt it realizes inwardly its own murderous tendencies. As we have seen, regression to the sadistic-anal phase was the motive for the transformation of the symptoms in the first case. In the *last* case the change of symptoms took place after both the hate-tendencies and the severity of the super-ego had been modified by the favourable conditions of the transference.

This material, acquired by the observation of cases, enables us to explain as follows the relation of agoraphobia to hysteria on the one hand and obsessional neurosis on the other. We know from Freud that phobias must be classed under the heading of hysteria because they belong to the genital phase. The individuals in whom they occur seem to be regularly persons in whom the conflict of ambivalence is more acute and the sadistic tendencies are more severe than is usually characteristic of the genital level. The fact that the subject has attained to and kept his footing on that level probably prevents the formation of obsessional symptoms, but there is nevertheless a pull from the sadistic-anal level, which may give an impetus in the direction of regression and may produce either a metamorphosis of the hysterical neurosis into obsessional neurosis (as in Case I) or a fluctuation of the symptoms between the two.

Under certain conditions repressed impulses become mobilized and the relation to the tenderly loved object is regressively degraded to the identification with it which was once established and fixed. The aggressive impulses against this object, when mobilized under the same conditions, are turned against the ego (because of the identification) in a manner which threatens its very life.

The process reminds us of that in melancholia. There the object is introjected and its fate – the threat of death and the reaction of anxiety in the imperilled ego – is through the destructive instinct inflicted upon the subject's own ego. The difference is that in phobias identification takes place at a higher level of libidinal development and hence is transitory and can be corrected. It occurs only under special conditions and may be cancelled if the patient meets with response from, has access to and receives love from the love-object. The same applies to the inclination to aggression. If the object is present and affords protection this tendency, which otherwise jeopardizes the life of the subject's own ego, is cancelled.

My conclusion is that the characteristic feature of agoraphobia is that between the subject and the object against whom the hostile tendencies are directed an identification takes place under conditions inherent in the Oedipus constellation. The sense of guilt is appeased by the fact that in the 'turning against the ego' the latter comes under the threat of death. But the tension between the ego and the menacing super-ego is relaxed only when the presence of the protective love-object gives the assurance that that object is not in peril of its life and has not abandoned the anxiety-ridden ego.

In the last case which I described we were able to trace exactly in the transference the genesis of this tension between ego and super-ego. It came into play between the two aspects of the identification. In the one the subject identified herself with the degraded love-object and did so by means of the dangerous instinctual tendencies: 'I am like you and it is my instincts which make me like you.' In the other she identified herself with the severe love-object who prohibited gratification of instinct (the ascetic mother). But always this severity made itself felt *only* in the situation of temptation – in the street. Since my patients were women the first identification bore the mark of the feminine-masochistic attitude.

An important secondary symptom which I observed in these cases was a strong exhibitionistic tendency. For instance, my last patient was much freer from anxiety if she closed her eyes in the street. I discovered that there was an important central significance in passive and active birth-phantasies. In these, the idea of being 'away from home' and 'outside in the world' has an important symbolical meaning.

The dread of parturition, as an element in feminine-masochistic phantasy, is a direct successor to the dread of castration. It was precisely the cases of agoraphobia which made clear to me something that I think is characteristic of feminine libidinal development. The surrender of the desire for the penis passes straight into the obscure desire for a painful assault. Thus the castration-wish and its direct successor, the wish for defloration or parturition, have the same representatives in the unconscious of women. In them the dread of castration, when it is not mastered, is transformed into neurotic dread of defloration or parturition.[5] The process of metamorphosis can be clearly traced in the analysis of patients suffering from agoraphobia.

I have, moreover, an impression that feminine-masochistic birth-phantasies play the same part in male patients with this neurosis.

I do not know whether these cases afford a complete explanation of the problem why agoraphobia occurs only in the street. Of course, these patients must always have a tendency to anxiety, which breaks out under certain conditions associated with the street. Freud holds that these conditions are (a) the loss of the protective shelter of the house and (b) the temptations of the street. Temptation arises there when regressive factors have degraded the love-life into prostitutes and this is brought about above all by the masochistic tendencies so clearly manifested in my patients. Similarly, the street constitutes a special danger to exhibitionistic impulses, and these too were markedly present in the cases I analysed.

An important determinant was, I found, the passive and active birth-phantasy. Undoubtedly, too, the strong, libidinal significance (which Abraham pointed out) of walking and of the legs plays a secondary part in the whole picture.

Notes

1 Originally printed in the *International Journal of Psychoanalysis*, volume 10, pages 51–69, 1929.
2 Alexander, Psychoanalyse der Gesamtpersönlichkeit. Internationaler Psychoanalytischer Verlag.
3 This kind of anxiety formation is one of the most frequent forms of infantile neurosis, and we see it succeed very early in life to the anxiety due to separation from or longing for the beloved object or else blend with these emotions. The impression we receive is that the anxiety of 'longing' is followed by feelings of hostility and indignation against the faithless love-object who has deserted and abandoned the subject; the anxiety on that object's behalf is a condensation of longing with its positive feeling-tone and the reaction to the disappointment – a reaction negative in tone but concealed beneath the positive components. In a child this form of anxiety concerning a beloved object is the first sign that the conflict of ambivalence has set in. Now the problem is whether

this ambivalence is already a manifestation of the Oedipus complex or of a biological factor from which the child's first hostile attitude to the outside world results. In so far as the beloved object withdraws itself from the child and frustrates his libido, it becomes part of the hostile world around him. The Oedipus complex and the defusion of instincts which takes place when that complex passes would then reinforce and effect a neurotic stabilizing of the early infantile ambivalent attitude.

4 This kind of anxiety formation is one of the most frequent forms of infantile neurosis, and we see it succeed very early in life to the anxiety due to separation from or longing for the beloved object or else blend with these emotions. The impression we receive is that the anxiety of 'longing' is followed by feelings of hostility and indignation against the faithless love-object who has deserted and abandoned the subject; the anxiety on that object's behalf is a condensation of longing with its positive feeling-tone and the reaction to the disappointment – a reaction negative in tone but concealed beneath the positive components. In a child this form of anxiety concerning a beloved object is the first sign that the conflict of ambivalence has set in. Now the problem is whether this ambivalence is already a manifestation of the Oedipus complex or of a biological factor from which the child's first hostile attitude to the outside world results. In so far as the beloved object withdraws itself from the child and frustrates his libido, it becomes part of the hostile world around him. The Oedipus complex and the defusion of instincts which takes place when that complex passes would then reinforce and effect a neurotic stabilizing of the early infantile ambivalent attitude.

5 In a paper on 'Frigidity', shortly to be published, I will discuss these processes in greater detail.

Chapter 2

Claustrophobia[1]

Bertram Lewin[2]

SUMMARY

In 'Claustrophobia', Lewin references Edgar Allan Poe's 'The Pit and the Pen-dulum' (1842), evoking the type of claustrophobic fantasy (and imagery) of the dread of being caught and crushed by the gradual closing in of surrounding space.

In this short and rich paper (1935), Lewin briefly references the theories of claustrophobia from the 1900s as morbid fear and hysteria anxiety of being buried alive or shut in an enclosed space (Jones 1912; Ferenczi 1922) and ideas related to the wish and fear of being within one's mother.

Lewin, an American analyst, studied at the Berlin Psychoanalytic Institute (1925–1927). He attributes the aetiology of claustrophobic anxieties to the discoveries of Melanie Klein (1932) in her work with child patients and the analysis of their unconscious fantasy and terror of a *united couple* of mother and father engaged in intercourse inside the maternal body with a dread of expulsion by father's penis. Lewin praises Klein as the only analyst who answered Freud's question (1925) 'of what is the claustrophobic afraid?'

Lewin describes a female patient with an intrauterine fantasy of enclosure in the maternal body, feeling safe inside, without anxiety, until the penis threatens to touch her (and, by association, to destroy or push her outside). Anxiety appears only when threatened with the defence against claustrophobic anxiety of expulsion by the father's penis. This theory is later developed by John Steiner (Chapter 8) in his ground-breaking concept of 'psychic retreat' (1979).

He offers a second cause of claustrophobia, the threat of being born. In *Phobic Symptoms and Dream Interpretation* (1952, p. 203), he extends the theory of the claustrum to include agoraphobic anxiety as a defence against enclosure by projection onto open space of one's primitive fears. This concept was taken up by Henri Rey in 1979, in his seminal concept of there being no place of safety for the 'claustro-agoraphobic' person (Chapter 7).

Lewin's ideas of the child's curiosity and fantasies of birth, embryonic origin, and life in the uterus predate Money-Kyrle's classic papers: *Cognitive Development* (1968) and *The Aim of Psychoanalysis* (1971). In 1950 he argued that the claustrum fantasy arises in the actual nursing situation as the infantile 'oral triad': the wish to devour (eat), to be eaten, and to sleep.

DOI: 10.4324/9781003200284-2

Lewin emphasizes the prominence of skin and respiratory phenomena in foetal fantasies and their connection to claustrophobic anxieties of being inside the mother. The erotic skin and foetal breathing fantasies in intrauterine life are taken up by Esther Bick (Chapter 4), Frances Tustin, Albert Mason (Chapter 6), and Donald Meltzer (Chapter 5).

Lewin was influenced by Weiss's ideas (Weiss 1935, p. 67) of spatial components found in agoraphobia with uneven surfaces and the ground giving way (Lewin, p. 205).

Lewin's *Body as Phallus* (1933), *Sleep, the Mouth, and the Dream Screen* (1946), and *Addenda to the Theory of Oral Erotism* (1950) contribute further to the concepts of claustrophobia and agoraphobia.

TEXT

The technical term claustrophobia, introduced into medical literature by Raggi of Bologna in 1871, means literally a dread of being enclosed. There are several forms such a dread may take, and several fears that are akin to it, but current linguistic usage tends to limit the application of the term to a special type of fear dramatized for us by Poe in the Pit and the Pendulum – a fear of being caught or crushed by a gradual closing in of the space about one. This definition, which will be followed in the present essay, would exclude such fears as that of entering a closed space, which might if one wishes be considered "claustrophoboid"; but the reason for this strict definition will become clear as we proceed.

Claustrophobia is a type of morbid fear, a form of anxiety hysteria, yet despite the numerous detailed studies of anxiety hysteria to be found in the psychoanalytic literature, there are nevertheless few references concerning this particular phobia. Jones[3] in one place remarks that dreams and fantasies concerning one's own birth are very common especially in childhood and that these fantasies constitute the basis of such phobias as being buried alive or being shut in an enclosed space (i.e., claustrophobia) and many others. Ferenczi[4] too refers to the association between claustrophobia and the idea of being within one's mother: "The psychoanalysis of numerous dreams and of neurotic claustrophobia explains the fear of being buried alive as the transformation into dread of the wish to return to the womb." Elsewhere Ferenczi[5] states that claustrophobia and a fear of being alone in any closed room in one of his patients developed from an attempt to overcome masturbation. These valuable comments establish for us a relationship between manifest claustrophobia and latent fantasies of being within the mother's body, but so far no author (except Melanie Klein in passing) has considered the *specific* anxiety in claustrophobia, as this phrase is defined by Freud in *Hemmung, Symptom und Angst*. The question, of what is the claustrophobic afraid? has not been adequately answered. This essay will attempt to answer this question, in terms of specific anxiety and specific measures of defense.

A young woman of thirty had ordered her life in general so as to escape marriage and the male sex. A business woman, she affected masculine ways and consorted almost exclusively with women. For sexual pleasure she masturbated or, occasionally and casually, engaged in mutual masturbation with another woman. Men were often interested in her, for she was good-looking, clever, and wealthy, but with the remote approach of an intimate relationship they would find themselves baffled by alternations in her of tense moodiness and inept sudden aggressiveness; they would find her unaccountable and give her up as a bad job. Twice this patient had severe attacks of claustrophobia. One of these was in her berth on a sleeping car. She was on her way to spend some time with a married friend. This friend's husband had once caressed her, and it was while returning from the dressing room at the end of the car that the patient thought of this particular matter and felt a certain expectancy at seeing him again. Lying in her berth then she heard a man's footsteps as he passed by, and she was seized by fear. Subjectively this fear was marked by the feeling that the walls of the berth were closing in on her, by inability to catch her breath, by an intense warmth accompanied by sudden perspiration. She cut the attack short by jumping up and running into the dressing room. Her other claustrophobic attack occurred while she was spending some time at a friend's country place. A young man had been invited there without her knowledge to meet her, and it was while in bed that she experienced the same fear as on the train.

The analysis of these two incidents was accompanied by several interesting "transference phenomena" and transient symptoms. Thus she stated that she felt enveloped in an armor which the analyst's voice could not penetrate, then suddenly in terror exclaimed sharply, "Don't touch me!" While she was on the couch, the analyst was accidentally called out of the room and returning found her lying flexed on one side in the so-called foetal posture. It was learned that she had rearranged the furnishings of her two-room apartment: all the things in the sitting room that possessed any emotional value for her, excepting her piano, which was too large, – her books, pictures, desk and the rest, were crammed into her bedroom, and there she read or worked cozily in bed, with all her prized belongings crowded about her.

The terror of being touched appeared then in her dreams. In one of these a man identifiable as the analyst kicked a boat lying in drydock, which then plunged forward into the water. In another dream a long pole was violently pushed through a window pane into the room where she was lying; she grasped the pole in alarm and tried to pull it away from the man who was pushing it in. It became evident that the patient was imagining herself a foetus in the maternal body – but this idea itself did not cause anxiety. Indeed, on the contrary, this was an idea of safety or defense. The anxiety arose when the defensive wall was threatened, that is to say, when the penis entered or threatened to touch her. This case therefore answers one aspect of the question posed above as to what it is that the claustrophobic fears. The intrauterine fantasy is one of defense (flight) and relief from anxiety; the anxiety arises with the idea of being disturbed or dislodged by the father or father's penis.

A second anxiety situation arises when the intracorporal status is interrupted by the fantasy of being born. The patient described above, after being comfortably settled in her bedroom and after becoming aware of her conflict and what it was she was fleeing, decided to come out. This she did symbolically by moving her belongings back into her sitting room, to the accompaniment of typical dreams of being born, needless to relate here, from which she would awake in anxiety; and at the level of the current situation, after this symbolical rearrangement, she was able to make a psychological rearrangement as well. She entered her first love affair and was deflorated at her next menstruation.

Briefly then this case showed that the idea of being a child within the mother is a defense fantasy, and that while this idea is sustained there is no anxiety. The anxiety appears linked to one of two contingencies: The first of these is of being dislodged or disturbed by parental coitus, by the father's penis or by his pressure on the mother's body (and it is this latter version that determines the central claustrophobic symptoms we would call classical); or of being born. This second idea – of birth – has numerous connotations and is sometimes reducible to the first situation according to the fantastic tocology: I am being forced out of mother by father's pushing on her abdomen.

In the case under discussion, the birth process was supposed to be started by the father according to the enema principle: father in coitus urinates into mother's anus and the mother expelling the urine flushes the child out with it. (A variant of this idea has the mother bursting open from being overfilled with water.)

The infantile material in this patient concerned an observation of parental intercourse (reconstructed from screen memories) and memories of her mother's pregnancy and the birth of a sibling when the patient was three years old. Early masturbation was accompanied by ideas of parental coitus with herself in the uterus. Obviously, some information concerning coitus and pregnancy is needed to give rise to such fantasies. During her analysis then, the fear of a male approach reactivated the fears attaching to these early fantasies. Dr. Monroe A. Meyer has told me of a case of true claustrophobia in which it was found that as a child the patient had actually retired into enclosed spaces to masturbate; I should interpret this as probably an acting out of the ideas referred to above.

In another case a puberty claustrophobia was combined with a fear of going blind. This patient slept for many years in the parental bedroom, was constantly present at, and aware of, parental intercourse, and barely missed witnessing the birth of a younger child. The patient's anxiety attacks were especially marked by an attendant almost asthmatic difficulty in breathing, and it was from her that I learned an interesting theory of how a baby breathes while it is in the mother's body. The baby lies in the body immersed in water. When the mother urinates the water is partly drained off and its level sinks. The baby's head floats at the top, like the bell float in an old-fashioned water-closet tank. The water-closet tank, indeed, suggested the theory.

The baby's head comes up as it were for air, the baby inhales, and as in the tank the water gradually rises and immerses the head again completely. Another patient came upon precisely the same idea, which played an important role in furnishing the latent content for early anxiety dreams. In these dreams the patient was under water rising to the surface, but her head always met the bottom of a boat or some structure that prevented its coming to the surface. The later neurosis of this patient, which unfortunately cannot be reported, affected chiefly the respiratory function.

The questions that arise in the child's mind concerning the embryo, its origin and physiology, its life in the uterus, and the cause of its ultimate birth, with the infantile and childhood theories designed to answer these questions leave their mark in fantasy, dream and symptom. In the illustrations given above I have pointed out the prominence of skin and respiratory phenomena attending the fantasy of being a foetus. Skin and chest sensations are particularly prominent in claustrophobic anxiety. Several analytic observers have been struck by the erotic skin and respiratory phenomena of early infancy and some have speculated on intrauterine libido organizations dominated by the skin or by the apnoeic respiratory tract. Aside from this, however, there is no doubt about the prominence of these two fields in connection with the *fantasy* of being in the mother, and they are bound up with ideas concerning the tactile sensations and the breathing of the foetus.

The process which initiates the fantasy of being in the mother's body is the familiar one of partial identification through oral incorporation. In several instances the fantasy was preceded by active oral aggression. This was true historically in the case reported at the beginning of this paper, where the mother's pregnancy led the three-year-old girl to bite everything and everybody in tantrum-like rages. The latent wish is to bite or destroy the foetus by an oral attack. The fantasy gratification of this wish leads to an identification with the foetus, thought of as a quasi-part of the mother's body. In some instances of this identification process, a checking of the oral-sadistic wish led to its reversal into the opposite, – that is, a wish to be eaten by the mother, but with the same consequences, for after being ingested the wisher found himself in the mother's body in place of the foetus. In one case this reversal was indicated in a series of dreams, in the first of which coitus with the pregnant woman was undertaken with a "biting penis", a snake, later with a rat; finally after the reversal, by means of a cucumber, which disappeared for good. In an interesting footnote in her book *The Psychoanalysis of Children* (p. 329), Melanie Klein remarks that claustrophobic anxiety, in some forms, appears to be connected with the idea of being shut up within the mother, which may be then deflected and limited to the genital, so that it consists in a fear of being unable to disengage the penis. She relates this to the infantile fear of both parents united in coitus and of being castrated by the father's penis in the mother's body. This finding would not be at variance with the ideas put forward in my account, namely, that the entrance into the mother is conceived as an eating or a being eaten. Indeed fantasies of entering the mother through some other portal than the mouth are quite probably distortions of this one.

The central claustrophobic fantasy according to the definition we are using is the fear of being expelled from the mother's body by the crushing, flushing, or other activity of the father. From this would radiate certain other combinations of ideas concerning coitus and the mother's body that would give rise to related fears. Thus, the fear of entering an enclosed space, as in the case reported by Oberndorf,[6] has among its latent ideas the one that the enclosure is the mother's body; however, the person who fears to enter does not identify himself with a foetus but with a phallus. Yet the underlying dynamics are very similar, for the identification with the foetus or with the penis is of the same sort, – an identification of the person's body with a part (or quasi-part) of another person through a fantasied oral ingestion of this part. The identification of one's self with the penis may instructively be compared with the identification with a foetus. Both originate through an oral incorporation of the "part" and the ensuing identification with it.[7] But the penis and its functions are well known, whereas the foetus and its behaviour, how it lives and breathes, are in the main unknown and only to be guessed at by the inquisitive child. Thus it is that in contrast with the almost uniform ideas concerning the penis and what it can do, the ideas as to what the foetus is like and what the foetus can do are very diverse.

Claustrophobic anxiety, to summarize, is correlated with the idea of being disturbed while an embryo in the mother's body, especially by parental coitus. The antecedent of the fantasy of being a foetus is an oral aggression against a real foetus, which leads to an incorporation of and identification with the foetus, the incorporation and identification being of the type known as "partial"; and the fantasy takes its form and ideational content from early childhood theories of gestation, embryology and birth.

Notes

1 Read before the Thirteenth International Psychoanalytic Congress at Lucerne, 1934.
2 Originally printed in the *Psychoanalytic Quarterly,* vol. 4, pp. 227–233.
3 Jones, Ernest: *Papers on Psychoanalysis,* p. 256.
4 Ferenczi, Sándor: *Further Contributions,* etc., p. 357.
5 Ferenczi, Sándor: *Contributions to Psychoanalysis*, p. 51.
6 Oberndorf, Clarence P.: Analysis of a Claustrophobia. Medical Record, 1915.
7 See Lewin, Bertram D.: The Body as Phallus. *Psychoanalytic Quarterly*, Vol. II, 1933.

References

Ferenczi, S. (1994 [1922]). Bridge Symbolism and the Don Juan Legend. In *Further Contributions to the Theory and Technique of Psychoanalysis* (pp. 356–358). Karnac.
Freud, S. (1925). Inhibitions, Symptoms, and Anxiety. In *SE* (Vol. 20). Hogarth Press, 1953–1974.
Jones, E. (1912). Letter from Ernest Jones to Sigmund Freud, May 7, 1912. *The Complete Correspondence of Sigmund Freud and Ernest Jones 1908–1939.* 28:139–140.
Klein, M. (1932). The Psycho-Analysis of Children. *The Psycho-Analysis of Children.* 22:1–379.
Lewin, B. (1933). Body as Phallus. *Psychoanalytic Quarterly.* 2:24–47.
Lewin, B. (1946). *Sleep, the Mouth, and the Dream Screen. Psychoanalytic Quarterly.* 15:419–434.

Lewin, B. (1950) Addenda to the Theory of Oral Erotism. In *The Psychoanalysis of Elation*. Norton.

Lewin, B. (1952). Phobic Symptoms and Dream Interpretation. *Psychoanalytic Quarterly*. 21:295–322.

Money-Kyrle, R. (1968). Cognitive Development. *International Journal of Psychoanalysis*. 49:691–698.

Money-Kyrle, R. (1971). The Aim of Psychoanalysis. *International Journal of Psychoanalysis*. 52:103–106.

Poe, E.A. (2013 [1842]). *The Pit and the Pendulum*. Penguin Classics.

Steiner, J. (1993). *Psychic Retreats: a clinical illustration, Chapter 2. Psychic Retreats: Pathological Organizations in Psychotic, Neurotic and Borderline Patients*. Routledge, pp. 14–39.

Weiss, E. (1935). Agoraphobia and Its Relation to Hysterical Attacks and to Traumas. *International Journal of Psychoanalysis*. 16:59–83.

Chapter 3

Agoraphobia and Its Relation to Hysterical Attacks and to Traumas[1]

Edoardo Weiss[2]

SUMMARY

Edoardo Weiss was an Italian analyst and ego psychologist influenced by Freud and his mentor, Paul Federn.

Weiss regards claustrophobia and agoraphobia as an *intra-ego* conflict with the inverse relationship representing the unconscious fear of confinement inside of, or expulsion from, the primal body space of the maternal womb. The agoraphobe seeks confinement to avoid outdoor, open spaces when his ego is in fear of losing control over the repressed drives (Agoraphobia in the Light of Ego Psychology, p. 4). The dread of agoraphobia – of open places – signifies the 'empty spaces' of the castrated mother with a missing penis (Weiss, 1935). The theme of spatial confinement in the claustro-agoraphobic dilemma is developed further in Chapters 7 and 8, by Henri Rey (1979) and John Steiner (1993).

Agreeing with his predecessor, Helene Deutsch, Weiss describes two types of agoraphobes, both suffering from internal dangers: those who project their anxieties into external objects or situations, which he refers to as 'projection phobias', and those who suffer from internal dangers caused by unconscious psychic conflict (Federn's Ego Psychology and Its Application to Agoraphobia ([1953] 1:614–628).

Melanie Klein attributed Weiss as coining the term 'projective identification' in 1925 (*The Psychoanalysis of Children* [1932], p. 250). One can sense Weiss's influence on Klein in her exploration of excessive projective identification and the invasive occupation of the object's mind (Klein, 1955). Weiss describes ego distortion between where oneself ends and the external world begins (1953, p. 624), leaving the agoraphobe without shape and feeling lost in space (ibid., p. 624).

Weiss believes that agoraphobic anxiety is caused by the trauma of early object loss and helplessness in interpersonal relationships. He describes the role of emotional development in agoraphobia as related to prematurely leaving the mother and super-ego pressure from the father to grow up. The concept of pseudo-maturity is later seen in the work of Meltzer in Chapter 5 (Meltzer, 1966, 1967, 1973, 1986, 1990).

DOI: 10.4324/9781003200284-3

Weiss's contributions to agoraphobia, depersonalization, identity diffusion, boundary loss, and bodily spatial distortion are reflected in the work of Henri Rey's (Chapter 7) description of marsupial space. He likely influenced Mervyn Glasser's formulation of the 'core complex', where Glasser describes a patient as 'imagining himself crawling up the birth canal and snuggling up inside the womb', knowing 'what it must feel like to be a chicken in an egg, wanting to burst out of its confining, suffocating shell' (Glasser, 1979, p. 164). Weiss may have influenced Winnicott's concept of the maternal environment and primitive emotional development (Winnicott, 1945, 1949, 1953, 1963).

TEXT

The analyses of a traumatic neurosis and of some twenty cases of agoraphobia and similar phobias have led me to conclude that there is an intimate connection between three separate problems: the significance of hysterical attacks, of psychic traumas and of the anxiety experienced in agoraphobia, which I take as a typical example of the mechanism of phobias in general.

I

Freud[3] originally defined the hysterical attack as 'nothing but phantasies projected and translated into motor activity and represented in pantomime'. These phantasies are, as he tells us, unconscious and, like the latent dream-thoughts, subject to distortion, a process which comprises condensation, multiple identification, antagonistic inversion of the innervations and reversal of the sequence of events. Freud holds that the hysterical attack is a substitute for an autoerotic gratification, previously practised and since given up, and that the loss of consciousness, the '*absence*' characteristic of such attacks, 'is derived from the fleeting but unmistakable loss of consciousness which can be observed at the climax of every intensive . . . sexual gratification'. We know, further, the view taken by Freud of the phenomenon of the *arc de cercle*, characteristic of major hysterical attacks: he holds that it represents 'an energetic disavowal by antagonistic innervation of the position suitable for sexual intercourse'. Ten years ago I published an interpretation of the *arc de cercle*[4] which was suggested to me by a quite unequivocal dream related by a female patient. Freud himself tells us that dreams often contain the explanation of hysterical attacks. My patient, a hysteric, dreamt that she assumed the *arc de cercle* posture with the feeling that, in so doing, she was squeezing out something in the region of the clitoris, and in the dream she actually had the sensation of that organ's turning into a prominent excrescence. Her association to this was the expelling of fæces, and the excrescence suggested to her the penis. By means of the *arc de cercle* she changed from a concave (female) attitude to a convex, protruding (male) attitude. Her whole body took part in the action of pressing out the penis. The analogy with parturition is unmistakable.

Hence we can expand Freud's account of the *arc de cercle* as follows: her energetic disavowal of the position suitable for sexual intercourse – Freud is, of
course, referring by implication to the *female* attitude – is actually supported by
the acquisition of a penis. Nine years after I published this interpretation Radó[5]
worked out in considerable detail the notion of this phantasied penis, to which
he gave the name of 'wish-penis', and showed that it is a phantasy of universal
occurrence in women.

In the case which we are now considering it appears that the patient's sexual
aim was the acquisition of a penis. It appeared from her analysis that in childhood the discovery that she was (as she imagined) castrated led to her loss of any
possibility of genital gratification. When she assumed the *arc de cercle* posture,
she was making good the supposed defect. In her unconscious the possession of
a penis was essential for sexual gratification: the *arc de cercle* represented a displacement of her sexual aim on to the attainment of this essential condition.

The following is another very clear instance of this type of displacement. A certain woman was the mistress of a man whom she would have liked to marry. She
and her husband had obtained a divorce on grounds of childlessness. The man
with whom she had relations could not make up his mind to marry her, precisely
because he too wanted children. Her narcissism was bitterly mortified by her ste-
rility. She never arrived at complete orgasm with her lover, coitus merely producing in her strong sexual excitation. Intercourse began to be succeeded on every
occasion by a hysterical attack, in which she lost consciousness, complained of
abdominal pains and finally vomited. She then came to herself again with a sense
of well-being and relief. These hysterical attacks completed the sexual orgasm,
acting as a substitute for the consummation which had been lacking. They did
not, however, signify sexual intercourse but rather the state of pregnancy. She had
been prevented from arriving at sexual orgasm by her severe narcissistic mortification, which had reference originally to her lack of a penis and, secondarily,
to her childlessness. Just as in our first case, displacement of the sexual aim had
occurred, and what the patient was seeking was a phantasied reparation of the
psychic injury she had sustained.

A hysterical attack, however, does not always, as in the case of this woman,
bring about a discharge of the internal tension which has gradually accumulated.
On the contrary, while in some instances gratification ensues, in others this is not
so – indeed, the effect may be rather that of a fresh trauma.

Owing to the existence of a connection persisting in the unconscious between
libidinal discharge and the release of destructive forces, sexual impulses give rise
to destructive cathexes. In a hysterical attack, as in every attempt of the libido
to break through, a libidinal and a destructive impulse come into conflict. If the
effect upon the subject is in the nature of a shock or trauma, we conclude that the
death-instinct is the stronger of the two; if, on the other hand, a sense of relief
is experienced, we assume that the libido has gained the upper hand. We must
remember, however, that its victory often fails to conform with reality, as, for
instance, when a woman phantasies that she has acquired a penis.

Let me give an illustration of the difference between a traumatic hysterical attack and one which had the effect of liberation, both occurring in the same patient.

A girl of thirteen had an attack of the following kind nine months after her first menstrual period. During the recreation-hour at school she had hardly left the class-room when she was overcome by a feeling that she was turning into another person. She felt a tremendous change coming over herself and her surroundings, and this gave her an indescribable sense of horror. She fought against the feeling, being determined to retain her own ego, but she could not resist it, and her anxiety became so acute that, for a short time, she completely lost consciousness. When she came to herself, she heard herself give a loud scream. With this cry of extreme terror, the attack passed off, as though she had by that means orally expelled something from her inner being. She now found herself kneeling on the floor. She had also had a conscious dread that she might never return to her real self, and this was the most frightful element in the whole situation.

Subsequently, these attacks recurred frequently; sometimes she even had more than one in a day. At first, they came upon her at home as well as outside and were accompanied by an uncontrollable impulse to throw herself on the ground. Later, they only occurred out of doors and in the street. Her dread of their happening in the street or in some other public place made her afraid to leave the house, for going out was liable to bring on an attack. Although, as the years passed, these gradually became less frequent, her anxiety grew more and more acute and, in order to keep them at bay, she had to sacrifice her freedom of movement. In the end, she had almost given up going out at all, and led a life totally devoid of interest. She was in a constant state of depression, shut off from the outside world and without any hope of ever escaping from this condition of torment, which kept her a prisoner in the house and sometimes in her own room. It was about nine years after the onset of this phobia that she came to me to be analysed; in about two and a half years she had practically recovered.

Analysis showed that what the attacks really signified was the patient's identification with her mother in childbirth. She had an unconscious phantasy of taking her mother's place with her father in order to have a child by him. Birth was conceived of orally: in her childhood the patient (who had an unusually strong oral fixation) had really imagined that birth took place by the mouth. The extreme sense of depersonalization which overcame her in these attacks was determined by her deep identification with her mother and signified: 'It is not I myself; it is my mother'. The person whom she felt she turned into was called in the patient's mind 'Mary', though she did not know why: 'Mary' was her mother's second name. This change of identity, which she always feared might be permanent, also signified death, for, as a child, when her baby brother was born, she had wished that her mother might die, and now, in her identification with the latter, she felt herself confronted with the same fate, which was embodied in the dread of 'never coming to herself again'. Finally, certain dreams and associations showed quite clearly that the sense of change signified also mutilation, i.e. castration.

As the analysis progressed, the hysterical attacks ceased and the patient became much freer. It was not until two years had passed without any such disturbance that she was seized, during the analytic hour, with an attack of quite a new type. She retained full consciousness, but the muscles of her abdomen, thorax and throat underwent severe spasms, she exhibited the typical *globus hystericus*, coughed violently, as though to get rid of something in her throat, and rolled about on the sofa. I said to her that these new and harmless attacks were a guarantee that the former dreadful ones would not recur, whereupon she gave a laugh of delight, although she was still suffering from spasms. In fact, these became so violent that she nearly fell off the sofa and I had to go to the rescue. Thereupon she flung her arms round my neck, as though to steady herself, and for a time would not let me go. When the spasms occurred, she also slightly bit my finger. After this attack she had a sense of well-being and told me that, during it, she had experienced genital (vaginal) sensations.

The following night she dreamt that she had a second attack at my house, during analysis, and that she tried to bite my ear. In the dream she was conscious of purposely prolonging the attack in the hope that I would kiss her. Thus it was designed to secure sexual gratification. I explained to her about the epinosic gain and told her to give me her associations to the dream. Instead, however, she was seized with a similar, though less violent, attack. While it was still in progress, I again asked her to give her associations and she signed to me that one had come into her mind. When she was able to speak again, she told me that, during the attack, which she did not take excessively seriously, a fresh recollection had suddenly occurred to her: she recalled that, one of the first times she had an attack, she had been in the street with her father and had instinctively clutched at his penis for a moment. In the next few days of analysis, she became conscious of fellatio-phantasies and gave associations about the movements of the child in the womb, etc. Further associations, fresh recollections and the interpretations which I gave her (though indeed they were obvious) assisted her to become more and more normal sexually, and no more attacks have occurred.

The patient's first attacks terminated in nothing less than death and castration, but the final ones signified the attainment of sexual satisfaction: 'In the end I do get a penis from my father, and I conceive and bear him a child without having to pay the penalty of death.'

II

It is only natural that the ego should react with anxiety whenever it becomes aware of the imminence of an attack which will have traumatic effects. The attack itself represents the dreaded situation. In the case we have been considering the patient's anxiety had a conscious, as well as an unconscious, content: she dreaded consciously the repetition of a former hysterical attack, of the latent meaning of which she was unconscious. There are, however, internal traumatic experiences which the patient generally cannot put into words; he merely says that he feels dreadfully bad and has an oppressive sense of anxiety. In such cases the only noticeable feature is the anxiety and we speak simply of an anxiety-attack. But here too the anxiety actually relates to a psychic experience which is difficult to describe but is analogous to a hysterical attack. It is, however, confined to the emotional sphere of the ego and remains without motor expression. Patients of this type (in contrast to those suffering from true hysterical attacks) appear to focus their whole anxiety on these 'anxiety-attacks'. The internal experience which evokes them consists of the most distressing sensations, as various as the manifestations of hysterical attacks and, like the latter, psychologically determined. Many patients have a sense of alienation or complain of giddiness, while others cannot feel their legs when they walk, or else have strange sensations in them which they find it hard to describe: for instance, they say they feel as if the ground were giving way under their feet or as if they were walking on the verge of a precipice or on an uneven surface, etc.

How does the ego try to protect itself from the repetition of such internal traumatic experiences? Its strategy consists in avoiding everything which may help to evoke them and in finding all possible means of keeping them at bay. Hysterical sexual anæsthesia and the repression, which is its source, have long since, little by little, become established in these patients. Then, if the subject is faced with a *real* situation which stirs up in him an unconscious sexual phantasy, the libido, thus stimulated, breaks through, in spite of the powerfully cathected destructive impulse bound up with it. If the destructive cathexes prevail over the libidinal ones, the result is a shock such as I have described, and from that moment the ego goes in dread of all such external situations as may stimulate dangerous, unconscious, erotic phantasies or stir up ideas about their evil consequences. Usually, agoraphobia arises out of a so-called anxiety-attack or, more rarely, out of a traumatic hysterical attack or the anxiety which precedes this. Freud found that this anxiety really has reference to the evil consequences of yielding to the sexual temptation to which the subject is exposed in the street, especially if he goes out alone. In claustrophobia, on the other hand, solitude brings a temptation to masturbate, the punishment being castration. In the cases of agoraphobia which I have analysed, I have found that 'to go out', 'to leave the house' had three principal meanings. In the first place it means. 'I am emancipated, grown-up like my parents. I can do as I please. I am my own master. I am no longer in my parents' charge': situations involving exposure to sexual temptation. In the second place it means to display oneself in public, to exhibit oneself. And thirdly it is associated with the idea of detachment from maternal protection. This is why agoraphobia so often occurs as an accessory symptom in cases of extreme helplessness; there often occurs secondarily a regression to the period of infantile dependence on the mother – a regression due partly to the internal aggressive impulses, to which the patient feels exposed in many distressing conditions and from which he endeavours to shield himself.

Many of those who develop agoraphobia have lost either father or mother in childhood. Analysis shows, to be sure, that in these cases, besides this loss, there was another factor which contributed to their anxiety, namely, the fulfilment of their wishes for their parents' death. The sense of abandonment does not necessarily spring from the death of either parent, for there are many cases in which the patient, as a child, felt himself repulsed by his mother (or father) or thought that no attention was paid when he expressed his feelings or had something to say. From that time on, he deposed his parents from their throne in his mind and his trust in them was severely shaken.

Sometimes the manifest outbreak of an agoraphobia, which has been, so to speak, germinating under the surface, is determined by certain superficial factors, which Freud has always taken into consideration and upon which the school of Adler has concentrated its attention to the neglect of all deeper causes. Such a crisis occurs when life makes any heavy demand upon the patient's ego. Thus, agoraphobia often develops at a particular phase in his life when he is required to take a step forward in the direction of independence, e.g. when he passes from a lower to a higher school, comes to the end of his student-days or begins his professional career; in fact, whenever he is compelled by outward circumstances to feel himself more mature, more completely adult. If he succumbs to agoraphobia at such a time it indicates that his capacity for adapting himself to reality has broken down before his necessity for emancipating himself and, in actual fact, he gives the impression of having become a child again, unable to walk by himself or, to express it more accurately, unable to go through life alone. Abraham[6] gives an account of the psychogenesis of agoraphobia in a five-year-old child who wanted not to be a 'walking child' [*Spazierkind*] but an 'infant in arms' [*Mutterkind*].

The sense of alienation which often accompanies agoraphobia indicates a reluctance on the patient's part to accept reality. The aim of the destructive instinct here is to abandon the ego to an alien and unloving world.

What I have so far said by no means exhausts the varied significance of agoraphobia in individual cases. In female patients (for instance, in the case of traumatic hysterical attacks which I have related) I have often found that 'to go out alone, to go shopping, etc.' signified 'to be, or to take the place of, the mother'; what the daughter wanted above all was, of course, to take the mother's place with the father. This identification led to the introversion of the hostile impulses towards the mother: the patient need not necessarily have wished that her mother should die in the street, i.e. that she should never come back, as Helene Deutsch[7] suggests in her very interesting article on the subject. Her investigations revealed in agoraphobia a mechanism similar to that of the obsessional neurosis. There was a preliminary stage in which the patient was exaggeratedly anxious whenever her mother was late in coming home: the daughter had an unconscious wish that her mother might die in the street. Because of her identification she feared a similar fate for herself. Helene Deutsch states that, in her view, the characteristic feature of agoraphobia is this identification with the object of hostile impulses, an identification whose roots are in the Oedipus constellation. I myself found in another case that to the patient's mind to go down a street and, especially, through a tunnel, signified to penetrate into the vagina, and the meaning of her phobia was: 'I am castrated; I cannot force my way in; I can go no further', and at the same time her legs gave way under her. Another patient had an unconscious idea that walking on the ground, the earth, was equivalent to 'treading on her mother's body and killing the unborn child within'. For her wish was that she herself and not her mother should conceive by her father. It is clear, then, that, in addition to the threefold significance always attached to the situation of going out, walking in the street, etc., various other meanings may suggest themselves in the minds of individual patients.

Anything which affords actual or symbolical protection from the manifest danger anticipated serves to allay the patient's anxiety: the proximity of a doctor or chemist, for instance. Similarly, anything which symbolizes the repairing of or protection from the unconscious trauma augments his sense of confidence. On the other hand, chance details associated with former traumatic situations accentuate the condition of anxiety. It increases whenever something recalls the danger, and especially if the unconscious sexual temptation is stimulated. It may happen, for instance, that a woman may feel safer in an avenue of trees than in a street where there are none, or that she may acquire a sense of greater confidence when she wears a particular hat or dress, which for her symbolizes the penis. This means that she is still struggling with her castration complex.

One patient, whose principal anxiety related to large open squares (she could not endure great 'empty spaces'), once dreamt that the analyst had to have sexual intercourse with her, but to her deep disappointment it turned out that he had no penis: there was simply 'an empty space' where the penis should have been. (This was the patient's own expression: '*un vuoto*'.) He then changed into her mother, for whom it was normal to have an 'empty space' instead of the desired organ. This dream shows that *open places*, from the dread of which the term *agoraphobia* is derived, signify *the castrated mother*. Probably some inner urge prompts us to put a statue, an obelisk and, especially, a fountain in the middle of squares.

Many women suffer less from their phobia if they have a child with them. It has always been said that this is because they feel the child's presence a protection from temptation. This may be the case; but I have often found also that having a child with them acts as an instinctual gratification. The woman who has a child – a normal substitute for a penis in the sphere of reality – finds her narcissistic mortification assuaged. One of my male patients who suffered from agoraphobia could not go out without a walking-stick, but naturally he could not explain how it would help him in an emergency. Many orally fixated patients always take care to have something with them to eat in case of need, for they are afraid of suddenly turning faint with hunger.

A certain agoraphobic patient in Rome had an anxiety-attack in the busy Via Nazionale. He succeeded in reaching the building where the Fascist Exhibition was being held, and this set him day-dreaming. He phantasied that he had done great things for the Fascist cause and imagined the Duce clapping him on the shoulder in a commendatory way. As these thoughts passed through his mind, he suddenly realized that his anxiety had vanished, and he went on his way in good spirits and with head erect. In general, patients suffering from agoraphobia feel the need to devote themselves to, and be recognized by, some person in authority: a father-imago. They generally have a blind faith in such an imago; these are people who usually accept their convictions on authority. One of my patients had a large collection of photographs of the King, taken in every possible position, while another had a similar collection of photographs of the Duce. In rarer instances patients devote themselves to religion – the service of God the Father.

The other side of the picture is the exaggerated arrogance and inordinate self-will which characterize many women patients of this type: qualities which they contrive to hide under a genial manner or a show of modesty. There are others who make no such attempt at disguise. In analysing such women one has to be especially careful not to wound their pride.

One of my patients always felt he must give himself an enema after an anxiety-attack.

Another well-known characteristic of persons suffering from phobias is that they pay a great deal of attention to their underclothes, often giving as their reason the fact that they do not want to be disgraced if it should happen in an emergency that they had to be undressed. The patient, whose dream of the *arc de cercle* I have recounted, could not put on any garment which had to be buttoned or was even close-fitting, for she was haunted by a fear that, if she had an anxiety-attack, she would not be able to get out of her clothes quickly enough. Her garments were wide and loose and fastened with press-buttons only, and these had to be in front or at the side, in order that, if an emergency arose, she could undo them with a single tug. She took the same precautions about her shoes. Besides this, she always carried a pair of scissors, so as to be able to slit up her garments in a moment if some unexpected obstacle prevented her unfastening them quickly. In her anxiety-attacks she had never actually found herself obliged to undo her clothes. These she regarded consciously as suffocating objects, of which one must be able to get rid instantly if one felt very unwell. Unconsciously, however, this exceptionally proud patient could not endure having to conceal any bodily deficiency, i.e. the lack of a penis. I cannot say whether the birth-trauma also plays a part in this connection.

Once a patient succeeds in overcoming his sexual inhibition to the extent of achieving normal orgasm, the fact of having discharged his libido in safety will greatly relieve his anxiety. A patient of mine who suffered from agoraphobia experienced very strong, normal orgasm the first time he had intercourse, and the result was that, in his mind, he himself and the rest of the world took on a vividness, a distinctness, a beauty and a charm such as he had never known since childhood.

I can give another example of a similar experience. A young man of twenty-three was sitting comfortably in the stalls at a theatre, listening to *Tristan und Isolde*. During the duet in the second act he began to feel bored: it seemed as if it would never come to an end. (A sense of boredom and impatience often precedes a patient's first anxiety-attack.) Suddenly he felt horribly ill and was seized with acute anxiety. Pale and bathed in sweat, he could scarcely sit out the act, after which he took a taxi and went home. This attack was the beginning of agora-phobia. I had to go to him, as he was unable to leave the house. I discovered that anxiety about his health had deterred him from ever performing the sexual act. After about a fortnight, the following recollection came into consciousness. At the age of five or six he had seduced a little girl of the same age, with whom he used to play at circuses. During their games she had roused his sexual curiosity and he had induced her to masturbate with him in secret. Once, however, they were discovered and punished and he was never allowed to see his little friend again. I pointed out to him the connection between these experiences in his childhood and his anxiety-attack at the opera, but he was not much impressed by the idea. Presently, however, I received support from an unexpected quarter. One evening, two friends carried him off with them to a brothel, in spite of his anxiety. (This, by the way, seemed to have diminished.) Here, for the first time, he had an orgasm with a woman – an event at which even his parents were delighted. He thus dis-covered that discharge of libido not only did not injure his health but actually made him feel better, the unconscious reason being that he felt he would not be castrated even though he gave rein to his sexuality. He now lost all anxiety and would walk about the streets all day long. He discontinued his analysis. Sometime later I heard from him that he was going on well; after that I lost sight of him.

Generally, an improvement or recovery brought about by successful orgasm does not last long, unless this result has been attained by a thorough analysis. The following abbreviated case-history illustrates this point. A young girl, who was excessively proud and determined to secure freedom and independence, had a powerful masculinity complex but concealed it by her feminine charm. She fell passionately in love with a young man, who, however, rejected her advances. The result was severe narcissistic mortification. She was much too proud to make any further overtures, but repressed her deep love and felt that something within her was broken past mending, so that in all her life she could never love again. She thought she might very easily give herself to any man who asked her; in fact, to spite the man she had loved, she would have liked to lose her good name. This disappointment in love occurred just as she was about to enter the teaching profes-sion. One day, she went to the school for her final examination, and her mother went a little way with her and then said good-bye. Suddenly the girl was seized with a terrible anxiety-attack. She turned round and called out to her mother, who, however, did not hear her. The daughter had not even the strength to run after her but begged an unknown woman who was walking by to let her walk with her, as she felt so unwell. This was the outbreak of her agoraphobia. Her circumstances made it necessary for her to go on teaching, and for many years she suffered unspeakable torments from her phobia. Finally she met a man with whom she once more fell deeply in love, and this time her love was reciprocated. The pho-bia disappeared and she felt free: ready to do anything and go anywhere. But suddenly he deserted her in very much the same way as the first man had done. Perhaps she herself unconsciously provoked it. Forced once more by her bitterly wounded pride to repress her ardent love, she relapsed into agoraphobia.

Analysis showed that in this patient's case there was a constant repetition of the infantile mortification on account of her supposed castration, though the actual situation contributed to the content of her mortified feelings and their repression.

We must now consider what it is that determines the particular type of neurosis developed in cases of hysteria. In conversion-hysteria, as in other types, the castration complex always acts as a specific, ætiological factor, the patient having already attained (and repressed) the genital phase. Why then does an anxiety-hysteria develop in some cases and a conversion-hysteria in others? I cannot as yet answer this question, but there are certain points which I would suggest in connection with it.

When we examine more closely the anxiety-attacks characteristic of agoraphobia and similar phobias, we find that the patient's anxiety really has reference to a conversion-symptom – in a minority of cases to a (traumatic) hysterical attack and in the majority of cases to something analogous to this but confined to the sphere of affect. Thus we can distinguish two types of phobia. In the first the patient has a conscious dread of certain external objects or situations, because they are associated with external danger. For instance, animals, trains, fire, etc., may be objects of anxiety, because the patient fears the external consequences of situations connected with these. These phobias give the impression of real anxiety, exaggerated and irrational, and they are brought about by the projection of some instinctual danger. Agoraphobia, on the other hand, relates to an *inner* psychic state, a 'psychic conversion-symptom', and only indirectly to an external situation (being alone, walking in the street) which itself conjures up some other situation consciously recognized by the subject as an inner danger. Here the mechanism of projection is much less powerfully at work. There is frequently a resemblance between agoraphobia and hypochondria. Sometimes, too, we are reminded of the state of giddiness induced by heights: people who suffer in this way avoid dizzy elevations, so as not to be exposed to a psychic state which causes them distress and anxiety. We should be inclined to classify agoraphobia as a form of conversion-hysteria, were it not for one point which differentiates it from the 'true' forms of that disease: in agoraphobia the 'conversion-symptom' to which the anxiety relates is always short-lived, it occurs 'accidentally', whilst such symptoms as hysterical blindness or paralysis may persist for months or years. Evidently this difference is connected with the absence or presence of anxiety. That is to say, anxiety is an indication that the ego cannot tolerate a particular state or reconcile that state with its aims. This state must be concerned with the sphere of the psychic ego. If the latter is to remain intact, the (conversion-) symptom, which involves the ego itself, must be got rid of. In place of a persistent conversion-symptom the ego feels a persistent *threat* of one; the aim of the defence-system in a phobia is to prevent the occurrence and persistence of the disturbance of the ego. Bearing in mind the cases of hysterical confusion (hysterical amentia), in which there is generally a previous history of hysterical attacks, we shall conclude that there was perhaps a certain justification for the dread of the patient whose traumatic hysterical attacks I have described, that she might never come to herself again. In the same way we can understand why patients suffering from phobias sometimes fear that they will become insane.

To solve the economic problem of anxiety and psychic traumas we must consider it in connection with the ego's instinct of self-preservation. But what is the relation between this and the two primal instincts: Eros and the death-instinct? We must confess that, as yet, psycho-analysis has not found a satisfactory answer to this question: there is a large hiatus here in our theory of the instincts.

III

Let us now see whether our clinical data, taken in conjunction with our theoretical notions, will enable us to bridge the gap between the transference neuroses and the true traumatic neuroses.

We know from experience that the readiness with which an individual succumbs to a traumatic neurosis depends on the uncertainty of his psychic equilibrium even before the actual external trauma occurs – depends, that is to say, on the ease with which his destructive energy has been able to throw off the sway of the libido. The transference neuroses also are prefaced by a similar instability in the fusion of instincts. Here I would remind you that Abraham[8] in his discussion of locomotor anxiety conjectures that this symptom results from the repression of a keen, constitutional pleasure in muscular activity (pleasure in motion). At the time when Abraham was writing, the existence of the death-instinct and the way in which it is deflected into muscular activity had not yet been grasped. Pleasure in aggression was conceived of simply as negative libido. We are now in a position to understand more clearly the metapsychological aspect of Abraham's discoveries: with the calling-in of the reserves of aggression employed in muscular activity the destructive cathexes are reinforced.

We owe to Freud the discovery that one of the uses of libido is to turn the destructive energy outwards (e.g. in muscular activity) and so render it harmless for the ego. But this same energy, in conjunction with the libidinal cathexes, does also receive an outward direction in all those functions of the ego which have reference to the outside world (attention, perception, the process which we call volition, etc.), and it is precisely in this way that the subject masters that which lies outside him. This mastery through the extraversion of destructive energy, whether it be in the form of aggression or of possessive tendencies, also leads to the gratification of the libido, which often spends itself in pursuit of this aim of protecting the ego and strengthening its position in relation to the outside world. We see that this process constitutes a defence against stimuli. The libido's binding of destructive instinctual stimuli often amounts to its control of the destructive energy itself, which is then conducted along the channels indicated by the libido. One such leads to the establishing and maintaining of the harmonious synthetic unity of the ego. As yet we have no clear picture of how the libido masters the destructive energy; in fact, we do not even know what is the essential nature of psychic energy.

When a traumatic neurosis ensues from the breach of the external barrier against stimuli and the irruption of large quantities of stimuli, it is not these stimuli, penetrating, as they do, from without, which produce the after-effects. Examination of such cases shows that what really happens is that there is an increase or accession of *inner*, destructive, instinctual stimuli. This is what imparts to the situation its dangerous character. In my belief this actual accession of inner destructive energy, consequent upon the cessation of its extraversion, is the characteristic factor in the traumatic effects which follow upon such stimulation from without. I am supported in this view by Kardiner,[9] who, in an extremely interesting article on the bio-analysis of the epileptic reaction, draws attention to the sudden inhibition of certain of the principal functions of the ego – namely, those of the sensory-motor-perceptual apparatus – in true traumatic neuroses.

In such neuroses the sequence of events is, I believe, the following. The libido originally controls a certain quantity of destructive energy, binds it, is fused with it, directs it outward either in the form of aggression or, in the ego-functions, of perception, comprehension of the external world, muscular activity, attention, etc. Now, in the case of a trauma, large quantities of stimuli invade the ego, making such heavy claims upon it that it can no longer protect itself from the inner stimuli which, formerly, it was able to control (by repression or some other method). Thereupon, the latent neurosis breaks out.[10] Because of the greater demand made upon it the ego finds it more difficult to master the destructive stimuli which it formerly controlled: they slip, so to speak, through its fingers and act in a reflex manner. The earlier control of the inner destructive energies can be recovered only by an effort. As long as the ego fails to re-establish its mastery, it seems to an outsider as if the quantities of destructive stimuli, which made a temporary incursion from without, are continuing to act within. What has really happened is that the subject's aggressive tendencies, in their various manifestations, have been withdrawn and directed inwards. Thus it is that, after an accident, patients cannot trust their senses and have little or no power of concentration. I believe that the trembling so commonly observed in persons suffering from traumatic neurosis is, at least in part, due to the withdrawal of destructive energy from the muscular system. This appears to me to be the general mechanism of the traumatic neuroses.

I must state at this point that I am inclined to conjecture that the formation of the super-ego – which comprises the so-called 'internal continuation' of aggression originally sustained by the subject from without – is also the result of external traumatic factors which have brought about the introversion of his aggressive impulses. Here, it is true, we are concerned with the avoiding of a traumatic neurosis by finding a place in the psychic structure for the introjected enemies: the super-ego, that important component of our mental apparatus, has come into being. It is my opinion that this does not take place gradually but in a series of sudden developments, each consequent upon some trauma. This notion is in accordance with Freud's hypothesis that the slaying of the father provided the stimulus for the formation of the super-ego.

Aggressive impulses and attacks of rage in persons whose balance has been upset by a trauma may be construed as attempts to restore equilibrium by the extraversion of destructive energy. Similarly, the super-ego itself relaxes its severity when extraversion of such energy occurs in the form of aggression, as, for instance, when the patient has a negative transference to the analyst. One of the most familiar and striking features of neurosis consequent upon accident is the epinosic gain, which is responsible for the persistence of the neurotic disturbance. If a patient is absolutely compelled to fend for himself, e.g. by the stoppage of a pension which he has drawn on the grounds of an accident, his destructive energies are thereby forced to take an outward direction in the overcoming of external difficulties. In my view, the doing away with the effective epinosic gain is a valuable therapeutic expedient in the treatment of this type of neurosis, for such gain leaves him without any sort of incentive to extravert his destructive energies, and this is why it weighs so heavily in the balance.

There are certain transitional forms between the transference and the true traumatic neuroses. For instance, there are neuroses which do indeed ensue from an external trauma, but this latter has been brought about by the patient himself in fulfilment of some unconscious purpose. Here it is most obvious how a shock affects the existing mental equilibrium. The following is a good illustration. One of my women patients was knocked down by a motor, struck the back of her head on the pavement and was taken in a very agitated condition to a first-aid station. This accident had the following traumatic effect. Almost every night she had anxiety-dreams about it; she was afraid to go out alone and trembled with anxiety every time she had to cross the street, even when accompanied by another person, to whom she clung. She was terrified of being run over by a motor, not only when she saw one coming in the distance but even when there was none in sight, for, at first, she no longer trusted her own senses. She lost all her mastery over the external world, and felt that she could not sufficiently focus her attention upon it. At the same time she was tormented by a vivid visual impression of the striking of her head on the pavement. This memory was cathected with a quantity of energy which pertained to the death-instinct and had been withdrawn from her aggressive tendencies.

The accident occurred through a palpable parapraxis on the patient's part. She had been just about to cross the street when she saw a motor approaching at great speed. She intended to wait till it had passed, but the next instant she forgot this and prepared to cross just as the motor reached her and the chauffeur could not possibly avert the accident. This was a good illustration of what Federn[11] says about ego-feeling in connection with parapraxes.

I had already been treating this patient before the accident occurred. She came to me because she felt she must have some protection from her own self-destructive tendencies, which were a source of fear to her ego. Some years previously, she had made a semi-serious attempt to put an end to her life by bleeding to death, but she had soon repented of her action and felt very much humiliated by it. When she came to me, she was chiefly suffering from a craving for narcotics: she felt obliged always to take larger doses than she could tolerate. After a few months of analysis she was able to refrain from taking anything to make her sleep; then the motor-accident occurred. She associated with it the prostrating effect of the narcotics. She was conscious of a strong resemblance between the striking of her head on the ground and the stunned feeling which she used to have in her head as a result of the excessive doses which she had formerly taken. She had, moreover, dreams of men who tried to violate her and, even when awake, she took exaggerated precautions against this danger. Hence her parapraxis had the significance of being the victim of an act of sexual aggression and of committing suicide.

This patient's neurotic anxiety originally had reference to the inner danger to which her own destructive instinct exposed her, whether blended with libido in the form of masochism or in the form of destructive impulses pure and simple (if such do indeed exist). The parapraxis which led to the accident was a victory of this instinct over the ego's instinct of self-preservation. Thus we can distinguish two different factors which probably had a traumatic effect on the patient: first, the quantities of destructive stimuli from without, which made a breach in the external barrier against stimuli and could not be bound psychically, i.e. mastered by her; secondly, the victory of the inner tendencies to self-destruction. I may say in passing that, by means of analytical enlightenment (which had already helped her to some extent before the accident), the patient before long got over this trauma.

In this particular case the destructive instinct availed itself of an external situation in order to accomplish its purpose, at any rate in part. The traumatic experience left in the patient's mind a profound sense of the power and danger of that instinct and perhaps paved the way for its fulfilment. Her analysis showed, moreover, beyond all question that she had never got the better of the deep, narcissistic mortification sustained in childhood when she discovered, as she supposed, that she had been castrated. In both the intellectual and the moral sphere she had tried to find a substitute for the missing penis; such substitutes were, to use Radó's phrase, her wish-penises. An intellectual or moral failure denoted for her castration all over again. The original conflict was, it seems, being constantly reproduced, the conflict, that is, between the effort to secure the wished-for penis, in order to get rid of her mental pain over her castration, and the destructive impulse to castrate herself, inflict pain on herself, etc. At bottom, however, we have the eternal conflict between life and death, and it is to be noted that the ego puts up the greatest possible resistance to the death-instinct of the id and feels any partial gratification of that instinct to be painful.

Here is a second case, which can hardly be classified as a transitional type between the traumatic and the transference neurosis, although, as in the first case, a parapraxis on the patient's part led to unconscious self-injury (symbolizing castration). What we find here is a traumatic situation, revived by the subject's destructive instinctual energy in the post-pubertal period, because it was associated with a sexual temptation to which he must not yield.

A ten-year-old boy was just going to sharpen a pencil when the penknife shut up with a snap and one of his fingers was badly cut. The sight of the open wound (which hardly hurt him) and of the blood affected him very unpleasantly, and he suddenly fainted away. What distressed him most in the episode was not the sight of the cut but his psychic experiences when he was coming round again. Looking back upon it all many years later, he described his sensations, which had been repeated more than once in the interval, as follows. First there was a loud and most uncomfortable singing in the ears, of which he could never say just when it began . . . very faint, elusive and almost imperceptible dream-like feelings: dim, indistinct dream-images, such as one sees when one is falling asleep – human forms moving and passing like shadows, voices from a long way off . . . these dim and hazy dreams grew gradually clearer, and it then dawned on him that it was he himself who was experiencing all these sensations – previously he did not exist. The singing in his ears grew fainter and fainter and finally ceased. It was succeeded by an agonizing sense of disorientation: 'Had the whole thing been real and not simply a dream?' He felt quite weak, just as if he were paralysed, with all his strength gone and unable to help himself; he suffered indescribable torment and still was not sure of his own identity or how such a situation had arisen. Little by little he recollected what had happened just before he fainted, he no longer mistrusted the evidence of his senses, and his ego recovered its feeling of continuity. It was as if he came into harbour in a world which had seemed dream-like – even dimmer and more unreal than a dream – but which had in fact proved to be real.

The episode of the cut finger took place in the morning. At lunchtime on the same day the recollection of these traumatic impressions came over him and he was suddenly seized with the same feeling of faintness. He hardly had the strength to tell his mother that he was going to faint again . . . then he knew no more until he was once more coming to with the agonizing sensations he described. As is always the case with a psychic trauma, these impressions were too much for him: he could not repress them and, in spite of their extremely unpleasant character, they frequently recurred. He felt completely powerless and helpless with regard to his fainting-fits; they came on at the most unexpected moments, sometimes without any external cause. In this state how could he possibly go out alone? After two days, however, he recovered his confidence.

One evening, when he was seventeen years old, he was walking with a friend in a very busy street when he suddenly noticed that his sense of the reality of the outside world was forsaking him: the passers-by (many years later, in analysis, he recollected for the first time, two unknown girls who had passed him) seemed like figures in a dream or rather like the shadowy visions which haunt us when we are just falling asleep. In a lesser degree they were taking on the unreality which, on the occasion of the original trauma, had seemed to envelop the real people round about him when he came to from his fainting-fit. He was seized with acute anxiety: 'Am I going to faint?' he asked himself. This is an instance of what I have referred to as something analogous to a hysterical attack: it was accompanied by acute anxiety and it conjured up the agoraphobia from which the patient had suffered long before. He now became afraid to go out in the evening, i.e. at the time when one generally begins to feel sleepy. Sometimes, the fear extended to the day also and had reference especially to walking in crowded streets: he dreaded that he might faint and make a humiliating spectacle of himself before the passersby. He liked best to keep to very quiet streets or even to take refuge in a doorway where no one else was about. Curiously enough, this gave him a sense of security from his fainting-fits. One thing that is quite obvious here is the destructive constituent in the narcissistic mortification, in association with a libidinal, exhibitionistic tendency. As the result of analysis this patient made a complete recovery.

In connection with this case I would observe that, for a psychic trauma to occur, the subject must be conscious during the traumatic experience. Thus we see that the traumatic effect made itself felt only as the patient was gradually recovering consciousness after fainting. Further, we note that behind his dread of castration was the dread of aphanisis (Jones).[12] Fainting is *par excellence* a manifestation of the death-instinct.

IV

The analysis of the case I have described and of many other neuroses suggests certain theoretical conclusions which I will now briefly summarize.

According to Freud anxiety is a warning-signal of an impending traumatic state in the economic sense. When it is a question of 'real' anxiety, the subject dreads certain *external* destructive forces: it is stimuli of this sort that may upset our psychic economy. In traumatic neurosis, on the other hand, *internal*, destructive, instinctual stimuli are diverted from the channels in which they have hitherto been employed and continue the effects of the external stimuli which had formerly been operative. Freud recognized this state of things in his account of the aggressive operations of the super-ego, and he has shown how in the sense of guilt (dread of conscience) anxiety and the death-instinct are related. We now begin to see that in neurotic danger (i.e. instinctual danger) it is once more the destructive, instinctual stimuli which menace the personality. It is true, however, that this menace usually coincides with that of the super-ego.

Let us scrutinize more closely the mechanism of repression. Children are threatened with the punishment of castration (or one of its many equivalents) and with the withdrawal of the love of those around them, if they give way to certain impulses. The ego of the neurotic never loses sight of these dangers. Formerly, he anticipated them from without (at the hands of father, both parents, or other persons in authority); later, they have their source in the super-ego. To indulge in some particular gratification of instinct therefore is to expose the ego to danger (real or imaginary). Either the subject may suffer some act of aggression from without (or be abandoned, defenceless and unloved, to external destructive forces); or else he may fall a victim to the internal aggression of the super-ego, the continuation within, as it were, of the aggression from without. We know, however, that the true source of the super-ego's aggressiveness is the instinct-reservoir of the id, and that this aggressiveness derives its energy from the subject's own death-instinct, independently of the outside world. In neurotic anxiety (the dread of instinctual danger) the danger is, as I have stated, that of a possible traumatic state, resulting from the penetration of the inner barrier against stimuli by quantities of inner *destructive* stimuli, such as are inherent in the energic cathexes of the ideas of castration, the withdrawal of love, etc. We know that, when an instinct is repressed, what happens is this: at the cost of a certain expenditure of energy the subject keeps back the instinct on the other side of the internal barrier against stimuli, i.e. outside the ego, in order to avoid a trauma. The latter may, nevertheless, ensue, because these instinctual stimuli, alien as they now are to the ego, continue to make their way towards consciousness, and carry along with them self-destructive cathexes and thus upset the economy of the ego and paralyse the functioning of the pleasure-principle. (This is one of the distinctive characteristics of a psychic trauma.) In such a case we always find that there is a close connection between the idea of gratifying the instinct and that of the destructive consequences to be anticipated from its gratification. We are familiar with the fact that a repression is lifted when the ego's unconscious attitude to the supposedly dangerous elements is brought into consciousness and thus corrected, the cathexes of the death-instinct being thereby kept distinct from those of the libido. It seems that only the former make a breach in that internal barrier against stimuli which (to use a phrase of Freud's) separates and protects the ego from the foreign country within him. If the ego has not abandoned its repressive attitude, an invasion of it by the repressed instinctual stimuli may have a traumatic effect. For what they signify is the destruction of the subject's own person: 'I give birth and die in the act', or 'I attain to sexual intercourse and it degrades me to the position of a prostitute and an outcast', or 'I am raped, castrated', or 'I exhibit myself and thereby display my deficiencies, the lack of a penis'. Alexander[13] states that certain of his female patients who suffered from agoraphobia had phantasies of prostitution. Radó takes these to be derivatives of genital masochism; my own view is that the temptation relates to sexual discharge. The amplification 'to become a woman of the streets' is an utterance of the destructive instinct, announcing itself through the medium of the super-ego. It is an aggressive qualification on its part.

In all unsuccessful repression a libidinal impulse is at war with a self-destructive tendency; the victory of the latter has a traumatic effect. The anxiety experienced in phobia is a warning-signal of such a state of affairs: it is, as it were, a sense of impending death, a feeling which is probably the mode in which the traumatic state expresses itself psychically. What we are here dealing with is certainly not the mere dread of death: it is an actual process of destruction, emanating from the patient's own death-instinct (though generally inflicted indirectly through the agency of the super-ego), in which the ego becomes incapable of controlling the quantities of invading stimuli. It is easy to understand how such an internal shock can induce fainting. Thus agoraphobia may be regarded as a traumatic neurosis *sui generis*, that is, as an *internal* traumatic neurosis. By this I mean one in which the uncontrollable destructive influence does not assail the subject from without but is purely endogenic. I personally have never known such a neurosis to prove fatal, but about a year ago I read in an American newspaper that a man suffering from claustrophobia was imprisoned and, after having vainly implored to be released because of the intolerable agony his situation caused him, died in his cell 'from sheer terror'. If this case is correctly reported, we should account for it by saying that death ensued from endogenic instinctual aggression and that the man's anxiety was the psychic expression of, or reaction to, a severe trauma which terminated fatally.

The repression of instinct is an attempt on the part of the psychic apparatus to protect itself from the repetition of a trauma which it has already experienced; if, however, the repression is unsuccessful and the destructive instinct prevails, the trauma is thereby renewed. But, in my view, the victory of the destructive over the libidinal tendencies does not always involve the repetition of a trauma due to external stimuli. In many cases it produces on the subject for the first time an effect closely resembling that of a trauma but really resulting from the breaking through of the internal barrier against stimuli by the stimuli of his own destructive instinct. Here the function of repression was to prevent the traumatic influence from making itself felt at all, but, owing to the strength of the destructive instinct, the repressive forces have failed.

Radó[14] conjectures that in women the two conflicting elements are the wish for a penis and the pursuit of masochistic pleasure. In my own view, however, the crucial factor is not so much the latter as the death-instinct, whether its energy is fused in a greater or lesser degree with libido (and thus presents itself to the ego as a tendency to find pleasure in pain) or remains without any admixture of libido – if indeed this is possible. Masochism is probably a secondary phenomenon, arising, as Freud[15] states, from the attempt of the libido to render the death-instinct innocuous and follow where it leads: masochism presupposes the death-instinct. For if the destructive energy will not submit to the sway of the libido, as it does, for instance, when it is diverted into muscular activity, then the libido follows its lead, though it be only for a short distance. In fact, it sometimes happens that, in order to mobilize the libido at all, one has to drive it on after the instinct of destruction – and thus masochism develops. The ideational representative of the narcissistic mortification is cathected by the energy of the death-instinct and the reason why, in women, the dread of annihilation is most frequently embodied in their dread of castration or, as Radó puts it, of their own genital masochism is that their anxiety is suggested by their own anatomy: the structure of that part of the body which is most adapted for the orgastic discharge of libido. Yet behind this anxiety there lurks the dread of what Jones terms aphanisis, and this last underlies masculine castration-anxiety as well.

It may be objected that the death-instinct is a mere theoretical supposition and that it never occurs without some libidinal admixture, whilst masochism represents the clinical aspect of this primal instinct, blended as it invariably is in a greater or lesser degree with libido. But, even if it be assumed that the death-instinct is really never found except in conjunction with libido, it is, after all, only the destructive element in an instinct which can produce a traumatic effect and it is precisely the libidinal admixture which weakens that effect. So I do not think we are justified in speaking of a dread of the subject's own masochism (= the self-destructive tendency + libido). Just so, in chemistry, the action of a certain element may be studied in a compound, though it may be impossible to isolate it.

I have tried to show that Freud's hypothesis of the death-instinct, which was bound to revolutionize our metapsychological notions, throws considerable light on the mechanism of psychic trauma. And, further, that such traumas, to which Freud at first ascribed the greatest ætiological importance, must actually be given a place in the foreground of the picture. And, lastly, the conception we now have of the nature of a trauma enables us to trace a very considerable resemblance between the mechanism of the transference neuroses and that of the true traumatic neuroses, which has so long been a source of perplexity to us.

Notes

1 Based on a paper read at the Thirteenth Psycho-Analytical Congress, Lucerne, 1934, and published subsequently: *(1935). Int. J. Psychoanal. (16):59–83.*
2 *(1935). Int. J. Psychoanal. (16):59–83.*
3 'General Remarks on Hysterial Attacks' (1909), *Collected Papers*, Vol. II.
4 'Zum psychologischen Verständnis des arc de cercle', *Internationale Zeitschrift für Psychoanalyse*, Bd. X. 1924.
5 Die Kastrationsangst des Weibes, 1934.
6 'Zur Psychogenese der Strassenangst im Kindesalter', *Internationale Zeitschrift für Psychoanalyse*, Bd. I, 1913.
7 'The Genesis of Agoraphobia', *Int. J. Psychoanal.*, Vol. X, 1929.
8 'A Constitutional Basis of Locomotor Anxiety' (1913), *Selected Papers*, Chapter X.
9 *'The Bio-Analysis of the Epileptic Reaction'*, *The Psycho-Analytical Quarterly*, Vol. I, 1932.
10 There are, however, cases (not only of anxiety-hysteria, but also of paranoia and depression) in which external dangers are mistaken for dangers from within. The inner, destructive, instinctual stimuli give actuality to the inward reflections of external destructive forces.
11 'Das Ichgefühl bei den Fehlleistungen', *Imago*, Bd. XIX, 1933.
12 'The Early Development of Female Sexuality', *The International Journal of Psychoanalysis*, Vol. VIII, 1927.
13 Die Psychoanalyse der Gesamtpersönlichkeit, *Internationaler Psychoanalytischen Verlag*, 1927.
14 Die Psychoanalyse der Gesamtpersönlichkeit, *Internationaler Psychoanalytischen Verlag*, 1927.
15 The Economic Problem in Masochism (1924), *Collected Papers*, Vol. II.

References

Glasser, M. (1979). From the Analysis of a Transvestite. *International Review of Psychoanalysis*, 6: 163–173.
Klein, M. (1932). *The Psychoanalysis of Children*. Hogarth Press, p. 250.
Klein, M. (1955). The Psychoanalytic Play Technique. *American Journal of Orthopsychiatry*, 25(2):223–237.

Meltzer, D. (1966). The Relation of Anal Masturbation to Projective Identification. *International Journal of Psychoanalysis*, *47*:335–342.

Meltzer, D. (1967). *The Psycho-analytical Process. The Roland Harris Trust Library.* Great Britain.

Meltzer, D. (1973). *Sexual States of Mind.* Clunie Press.

Meltzer, D. (1986). *Studies in Extended Metapsychology. The Roland Harris Educational Trust.* Great Britain.

Meltzer, D. (1990). The Claustrum: An Investigation of Claustrophobic Phenomena. *The Claustrum: An Investigation of Claustrophobic Phenomena*, *144*:1–195.

Weiss, E. (1935). Agoraphobia and Its Relation to Hysterical Attacks and to Traumas. *International Journal of Psychoanalysis*, *16*:59–83.

Weiss, E. (1953). Federn's Ego Psychology and Its Application to Agoraphobia. *Journal of the American Psychoanalytic Association*, *1*:614–628.

Winnicott, D. (1945). Primitive Emotional Development. *International Journal of Psychoanalysis*, *26*:137–143.

Winnicott, D. (1949). Hate in the Counter-Transference. *International Journal of Psychoanalysis*, *30*:69–74.

Winnicott, D. (1953). Transitional Objects and Transitional Phenomena – A Study of the First Not-Me Possession. *International Journal of Psychoanalysis*, *34*:89–97.

Winnicott, D. (1963). Dependence in Infant Care, in Child Care, and in the Psycho-Analytic Setting. *International Journal of Psychoanalysis*, *44*:339–344.

Chapter 4

Anxieties Underlying Phobia of Sexual Intercourse in a Woman[1]

Esther Bick[2]

SUMMARY

Bick is best known for her theory of second skin (1968, 1986) as a primitive experience of the 'psychic' proto-mental function or ego boundary between mother and infant that contains the infant's early ego, preventing ego disintegration.

In this 1953 qualifying paper, Bick bridges the gap between Freud's drive theory and Klein's object relations theory. Bick incorporates the concepts of the dread of being buried alive and the concomitant fear of birth. Written after Klein (1935, 1940, 1946), Bick includes Kleinian object relations theory of the paranoid-schizoid, depressive positions, and projective identification.

Lewin's configuration of the infant's sensuous bodily experience, including intrauterine respiratory and early skin phenomena (Lewin 1933, 1935, 1952), is apparent in Bick's understanding of dynamics and enactment in analysis. Bick, following Deutsch (Chapter 1) and Weiss (Chapter 3), emphasizes the role of spatial dimensionality and compartmentalization in claustro-agoraphobia. Bick describes three claustra: the breast, womb, and head. Bick's patient uses the claustrum as a 'lavatory' for evacuation of unwanted parts. This concept is developed further by Bick's student and collaborator Donald Meltzer as 'toilet breast' (Meltzer, 1967). One intuits the influence of her supervisor, Bion (1962), in the theory of thinking and maternal containment.

In this chapter, we foresee Rosenfeld's concept of psychic islands, Steiner's concept of psychic retreats (Chapter 8), and Rey's elaboration of reparation and psychic repair of the internal object world in 'That Which Patients Bring to Analysis' (Rey, 1988).

Bick describes a frigid female patient with a fear of madness and an identification with a psychotic mother (and through projection, her analyst), who breaks down in the course of analysis. This patient experienced feeding at the breast as both nurturing and suffocating. Bick argues that catastrophic anxieties of destruction to the self and object underlie the patient's fear of sexual intercourse. Winnicott wrote a commentary on Bick's qualifying paper (Chapter 4), and one can recognize her influence on his paper 'Fear of Breakdown' (1963).

DOI: 10.4324/9781003200284-4

Hatred of the analyst due to the representation of psychic conflict and aware-ness echoes Deutsch's impressions (1929, p. 64). Both Bick and Mason (Chap-ter 6) caution the analyst against a premature interpretation of the root causes of claustro-agoraphobia, lest it elicits too much anxiety and induces a psychotic breakdown. Like Deutsch (Chapter 1) and Mason, Bick describes the intense 'watchfulness' through the eyes as paranoid control of the analyst.

Bick emphasizes the patient's fear of and guilt over the damage done or imag-ined to her internal objects, resulting in persecutory depression and regression. The desire to repair the damaged and dead actual parents from the destructive wishes to rob her mother's body and destroy the parental genitals contributes to her fear of pregnancy and intercourse. Similar unconscious phantasies are uncovered in the analyses of both Bick's and Deutsch's female patients who fear intercourse.

This article highlights Melanie Klein's child cases and Hesiod's world of mon-strous gods (Finkelstein, Chapter 9).

TEXT

My patient, a married woman now aged 37, was transferred to me five years ago after one-and-a-half years of analysis. Her complaints could be divided into four categories:

1   Claustrophobic fears of being trapped in underground trains, theatres, etc., on heights and on water, of being hemmed in by crowds, of being alone in the house and leaving it. Panicky fear of suffocation when she pulled a garment over her head and when she washed her hair.
2   Hypochondriacal fears and psychosomatic symptoms. Fear of losing her voice, her sight, her mind, of losing the power of her legs, of throwing herself out of the window. Frequent sore throats, choking and not being able to swal-low, breathlessness, colicky cutting pains, heaving.
3   Difficulties in object relationships particularly with women, feeling exploited, mocked and accused.
4   Inhibitions in work, eating, and intellectual inhibitions.

In appearance the patient is small, fair, neatly though plainly dressed, looks younger than her age. She comes from a small town, from a middle class family. Her father was described as quiet, reserved and reliable. Her mother, according to the patient, suffered from fears and complaints similar to her own, yet was the centre in company. The patient has a sister three years older who was described as bossy and bad-tempered in childhood, but now they are on friendly terms. My patient was born in 1916. Her mother told her that she was breast-fed for eight or nine months, that she was a healthy baby, and stressed particularly that she was quiet and did not cry. She talked early but was slow in starting to walk. When she was one year old her father was called up and posted abroad. He returned when my patient was about four-and-a-half. During her father's absence my patient slept with her mother and went with her everywhere. She was her mother's favourite whilst her sister was spoilt by her grandfather. After her father's return she clung to her sister who resented having to take her everywhere with her friends. This changed in adolescence. My patient had many friends, went to dances in contrast to her sister who was shy with strangers. When my patient was 21 her father died of peritonitis after a three days' illness, at the age of 51. Her mother had a nervous breakdown and the patient could not leave her. [In 1943 during World War Two] at the age of 27 she married a pilot three weeks before he was posted abroad. After their honeymoon she returned home. She went to stay with friends for a weekend but was called back by her sister because her mother had been taken ill. When she arrived in her mother's bedroom she found her dead. This was six weeks after the patient's marriage. She lived with her sister until her husband was demobbed in 1945. He went back to his old clerical job and since then they have been living in and near London. She described him as quiet, reliable and reserved like her father.

My patient felt she had always been nervous, had many fears but could cope with them. She thought she managed adequately during the first year of their married life in London – it later transpired that she had been ill most of the time with sore throats – but gradually the symptoms increased in their severity and she decided to get help from analysis. They bought a shop, which the patient ran, mainly to earn money for the analysis, and lived in a flat over it.

My patient was diagnosed as anxiety hysteria with phobic formations. When I began analysis in September 1948 the patient was 32 years old and had been married five years. I had no information regarding her sexual life. Very soon however when conflicts about sexual feelings apparent in her dreams were interpreted, she told me that she had never had intercourse. When I asked her about it she said they tried after they were married but she was too small, it hurt her. She was terrified it would shatter her inside and thought it was mad. It made her feel sick and it was not possible to go on. This information was given with the utmost reluctance and fear. Indeed during the one-and-a-half years of her first analysis no material referring to her sex life was obtained, nor was this a complaint she came to seek help for.

I am going to outline the outstanding features of the first two years of analysis at the end of which the patient suffered from an acute anxiety state, which she called her breakdown. I saw her four times a week. One of the striking characteristics of this phase was the intensity of [her] transference. From the beginning the patient started every session with remarks about my room but only about the part of it which she could see from the couch. The other part of the consulting room was never alluded to, though it was the first she saw on her way to the couch. She followed with intense watchfulness the minutest details in 'her' part and reacted with suspicion and fear to the smallest changes, e.g. when a book was removed to a different place on the same shelf or when one flower in the vase was at a different angle from the one of the previous day. She was acutely aware of any smells or sounds [such] as my breathing, smoking, moving, [and] the wind outside which she felt would break the tree. The smell of my soap reminded her of vomit and made her feel sick. When she could feel that there was no change in the room, no sound or smell, she felt relaxed and friendly.

Following transference interpretations the patient brought memories of the time when she was small and her mother left her to go to whist drives. She kept on pleading with her mother not to go. After her mother left, she lived in dread that something would happen to her mother. Once when she was three her mother left her outside a shop. This memory still haunted her. She felt plunged into a mad world, did not recognise anything. Similarly she was afraid something would happen to her husband if he did not arrive home punctually.

Another feature of this period was her total unawareness of her aggressive feelings. She saw herself [as] small, friendly, [and] wanting a fair share only, but [felt] victimised and humiliated for no reason now as in the past. Her mother exposed her to humiliation at school by not allowing her to play hockey and by making her wear liberty bodices. Her husband exposed her to the anger of her assistants and customers by not putting a match to the fire he had laid, and endlessly in this vein. When her assistants and customers accused her she felt petrified, [and] couldn't think, say or do anything.

She admired at times my large clean room and compared it with her crowded flat, which she could not keep clean. There were constant comparisons of flowers in my room, whether they were fresh or one of them drooping, well or carelessly arranged, whether they matched the vase they were in, in size, colour and shape. When the flowers were big a mad thought came to her mind, 'off with their heads', like in *Alice in Wonderland* and she felt terrified. There was one small vase containing small flowers, which she liked.

The gist of my interpretations of all the transference material was that she expressed through flowers etc. her feelings towards me, that she felt as dependent on me for her health and sanity as she did on her mother and husband. She reproached me for treating her carelessly as they did and making her ill. She felt she couldn't trust her positive feelings towards me because her admiration turned immediately into envy and jealousy, feelings she was most afraid of. Their power seemed to her so overwhelming because under their sway she felt herself to be the mad Queen of Hearts, cutting my head off with one thought in an offhand way. She felt then plunged into a mad world in which she neither recognised my headless body nor my cut-off head, standing for the cut-up body of her mother, a repetition of the haunting feelings outside the shop. She felt that there was one escape only from her mad world of fears, and this was when envy and jealousy were eliminated, when we fitted into each other like the small flowers into the small vase. The small flowers were standing for my nipple, the small vase for her mouth. She had to be the quiet mouth that did not cry and did not eject vomit and wind, I had to be the nipple that did not force itself into her, did not leave her and did not make her envious of the big flowers, standing for the big breast. The small flowers were also standing for the glans of the penis . . . which I had to fit into her small vagina without movement, i.e. penetration and without making her envious of the big penis of which it was part, perhaps like in intercourse with her husband. Whenever I interpreted her sexual feelings towards her husband she ignored it and when this was interpreted she felt she could not think or say anything, became confused and petrified. In fact the panic of intercourse was reproduced in which she felt I forced my interpretations, standing for the penis, into her.

She became gradually aware of the intensity and omnipotence of her sadistic impulses. An example: she was with her husband in bed and asked him to switch the wireless off. Time went on, she was boiling with rage but said quietly, 'It's getting late, switch it off'. She could have done it herself but was afraid that if she did she would scream and her scream would cut his head off. She felt now that she kept her husband like a dog on a leash and was terrified that he would leave her. Now she remembered how angry she was when in spite of her protests her mother was leaving her to enjoy herself. In phantasy she banged her head into her mother's stomach, strangled her, threw her on the floor, stamped her into the ground and exclaimed, 'So there!' She once remarked: 'I always kept my thoughts to myself, I thought they were mad.'

Another feature of this phase was the use of indirect language and the pattern of her dreams. My patient never expressed directly any of her feelings towards me . . . or any of her sexual feelings towards her husband. These were alluded to through flowers etc. as I have described. They were split off from her conscious communications, repressed and found expression in her dreams, which she brought to every session. The pattern of her dreams was fixed. They consisted of three parts. The first part represented intercourse fantasies in a hardly disguised manner, the following two were lavatory dreams. I should give an example later.

The predominant features of the first two years of analysis show the extensive use of splitting mechanisms similar to those described by Melanie Klein.[3] The patient split the room, standing for myself, unconsciously annihilating this part of me which did not belong to her. She split from her ego the aggressive self-asserting part and was left with a small tortured ego. Her sexual impulses were repressed and in the dreams the genital impulses were split off from the anal ones. In 'her' part of the room . . . she projected her split-off impulses and parts of the self and tried to control every movement of mine, lest I should force them back into her by sound, smell or musculature. Added to the splitting defences, projection, obsessional defences and repression, my patient used a particular defence of immobility in states of acute anxiety. In such states as I have described she could not think, say or do anything and felt paralysed. This aspect will be developed more fully in later material.

The patient could establish two types of relationship to me in the transference. Ordinarily she felt dependent but full of fear and suspicion. More rarely she felt free of fear but only on the condition that there was this perfect matching which I have described. This precarious relationship with me was constantly threatened. She had always to be on the alert, to watch, hear, smell, to predict my next movement. It necessitated the development of a faculty for clairvoyance, which she indeed achieved and produced telepathic phenomena of the kind Dr Gillespie [1953] described.

In the second year of analysis the patient felt some improvement on which, according to her, her husband commented. She described that she was no longer afraid of being alone in the house nor of sounds pursuing her when she walked upstairs, that she did not get angry over small things and was better able to cope with people. These improvements were not maintained owing to an accumulation of, to her, traumatic events which led to an acute anxiety state over the Christmas holidays. The symptoms of choking and breathlessness suddenly developed into attacks in which she felt she could not breathe at all. The events which intensified her anxieties were: (1) the Christmas holidays, (2) her husband's wish to volunteer for the Korean War, (3) the precipitating factor was an electricity power cut in her session, three days before the Christmas holidays, which cut off light and heat. The meaning of these events was highly over-determined. She felt that her chief protecting object, her husband, who mainly stood for her mother, was abandoning her in the same way as I was over the holidays. The power cut three days before my holidays repeated to the patient traumatic events in her life ending with the death of her father and mother. Her mother died *three weeks* after my patient's husband was posted abroad. She was terrified that her mother was buried alive because the doctor who signed the death certificate didn't go up to see her mother. She felt responsible for it and never told anyone of this fear. In the transference situation those events were repeated with me standing for her mother who was going to die. It was at the same time a repetition of her childhood situation when her father was posted abroad and she feared her mother's death. She had also felt responsible for her father's death. He died *three days* after an operation on a perforated appendix. She felt at the time she ought to have done something and blamed herself and the doctor. The meaning of the power cut in this context was that she was the doctor who cut my stomach and I had only three days to live. Immediately after the session of the power cut she had her first attack of breathlessness in a pub where she met her husband. He phoned me because she could not go home. I interpreted to her over the phone which relieved her anxieties for the time being and she came to the remaining three sessions.

During my holidays her husband phoned me that his wife had broken down completely. I saw her on the same day. When she came, she could not lie down, sat trembling and fighting for breath. I interpreted that she was afraid to lie down, because, as she could not breathe or speak, I might sign the death certificate on her like her mother's doctor and bury her alive. She quietened and told me of a most terrifying experience she had in the morning on waking. It was so frightening because she was sure she was not dreaming. She saw herself very small, clinging to her husband with her mouth and body. She felt she must get down or she would damage him irreparably, but knew that if she got down she would go mad and die. She could neither go on clinging nor get down and felt paralysed in agony. Her associations to clinging were 'a leash, no', she corrected, 'I mean a leech, a vampire'.

I interpreted that, through making her aware in the analysis that the leash with which she clung to me and her husband was her vampire mouth, she felt that I had made her more ill than before she came to me. The patient confirmed this. She had never been so ill in her life as in the last two days. She could not breathe, she could not drink at all because it choked her. She had to think about it all the time because if she stopped thinking she would stop breathing. She was afraid to be left alone for a moment and her husband had to stay away from work. She felt she could not fight any longer and wished to die.

The gist of my interpretations was that she relived and re-enacted in those two days the last days of her mother's life. The guilt over her mother's death was intensified because she felt that in going away for the weekend she left her mother to die alone. In her omnipotence of thoughts she felt she could stop her mother from dying as she felt she could stop herself from breathing. Added to this was the guilt towards the much-maligned sister, who had to carry the whole burden, not to leave her mother for a moment. She thus felt she alone would be responsible for her mother's death and therefore could not let her mother die inside her. This relation to her dying mother was internalised. She felt the dying mother inside herself and was identified with her – hence the fighting for breath, but she also was identified with her sister and therefore felt that she had to look after the dying mother, to think all the time in order to keep the breathing going. The internal situation was re-enacted with her husband.

The guilt . . . that imposed this task on her contained an accumulation of all her guilt feelings towards her mother reaching back to her relationship to the breast. The leash with which she clung to and controlled her objects was to her a symbol of her small mouth and body with which she felt she sucked the air and milk from her mother's breast. She took in this damaged breast which suffocated her from inside and could not feed her. She became aware that if she went on clinging, sucking, she would damage the only internal and external object that was barely alive and keeping her barely alive. She felt she must stop, because to torture any longer the good object would mean to become mad. She wished to die, but she could not die either because her mother inside her would die too. She felt paralysed in agony, held suspended, immobilised. We see here again the defence of immobility. It was a defence to her against the death of her protecting internal and external object and against the madness of the self. With this defence she attempted to suspend the disintegration of the good object and the self and to deny the death of the good object. In such states she felt she could neither take in nor give out. This disturbance of her introjective and projective processes made it imperative to her to regress from depression[4] into persecution. In the transference I became the mother, the sister, the husband who cut off the leash and let her suffocate, the doctor who signed the death certificate and cut the stomach. In addition I would think that the cutting of the leash also represented the cutting of the umbilical cord.

The inability either to breathe or to drink in her anxiety states shows the close connection between the two functions in my patient. Fenichel [1944], following

Oberndorf [1929], interpreted the fear of suffocation in claustrophobia as a reproduction of the infant's inability to manage its breathing while it drinks at the breast.
B[ertram] Lewin [1935] stresses the oral fears in claustrophobia and implies that
the breast is a claustrum.[5] Melanie Klein found that the inside of the body is felt
to be the enclosed space – the claustrum. The breast which suffocated my patient
from within was the internal breast claustrum containing the substances of the
object she felt she sucked out, the air and the milk. This breast claustrum she projected into two of her phobic symptoms:

1   The fear of being suffocated by the garment when she pulled it over her head,
     because she felt there was no air in it or bad air in it.
2   The fear of suffocation which she experienced when she put her head under
     the running water in washing her hair because she felt there was too much
     water or bad water. The water stood for milk.

As soon as the analysis was resumed, with five sessions, her husband could go to
work, but her increased claustrophobic symptoms remained. Except for analysis
she could not leave the house nor meet friends. She had no attacks of breathlessness in the sessions after the one I mentioned but she had them at home, on the
way to me, and acutely before she rang my door bell; once she was with me she
was free of them. From associations it emerged that she felt me to be the breast
penis, which protected her against her vampire mouth vagina impulses. A lavatory
dream of this period shows the link between breathing, urinating and defecating
and her genital impulses.

She dreamt that Prince Philip gave her perfume and then danced with her.
A young girl was cutting in between them. She didn't succeed and fainted. In the
next part she dreamt she wanted to 'spend a penny'. (This term referred to urina-
tion, defecation and the passing of flatus.) There was no lavatory, only smelly
holes cut in the ground. She was given two pills to dissolve and disinfect them,
but there were people standing about. In the third dream she was in another lavatory. A tin of disinfectant was hanging from the ceiling. She cut a hole in the tin,
became frightened and pushed the cut-out bit back, to hide it from the owner. She
felt full to bursting but could not go. She woke in fear with the sensation of bearing down. With this she meant that she was about to pass flatus. My patient had
difficulties for a long time in the analysis to give associations to her dreams. In
her wish to cooperate she went over them again. I treated the two lavatory dreams
as associations to the first genital one. To perfume which the Prince gave her,
the two pills she was given to disinfect her two lavatory holes, before she could
dance, i.e. have intercourse with him. To cutting in, she was the young girl who
cut out a hole in the tin representing both her father's penis and mother's breast.
She hoped it was done invisibly but was afraid that the owners would discover
it. She cut in between the dancing couple, standing for the parents in intercourse,
silently but did not succeed because her silent fainting made her rage obvious. It
was she who cut the holes into the ground standing for mother's breast and body,

filled them with flatus, urine and faeces, but again did not succeed because the smell gave her away. She felt full to bursting in all her lavatory dreams but on waking had only the need to pass flatus. This indicates that the cutting was mainly done with wind.

Reviewing the analysis so far described, together with the analysis of this lavatory dream, I would like to make the following comments. The two lavatory holes and the many holes in the ground stand for the openings in her body, which lead to the cavities in her body. The cavities are to her[6] lavatories filled with the cut-out and introjected bits of her mother's breast and body and the parental genitals in intercourse. In projection they became her claustra. Her first two lavatory holes were her mouth and her urethra and anus, which seemed to her to be one hole, a cloaca covered by the term 'spending a penny'. The picture that emerged in the transference, confirmed by her early history, is that the use of her mouth, [for] . . . oral elimination, was inhibited. She was a quiet baby who didn't cry. She felt that screams cut off the head, standing for the breast. Heaving is one of her symptoms and though she feels sick she cannot vomit because she is terrified of it. Thus she could not expel orally the winds, screams and smelly vomits. The cutting into the breast had to be done silently, invisibly, and without smells. This could only be done in quiet breathing. She started talking early. In her words were hidden the smells and the cutting flatus. The two intellectual inhibitions, spelling and decimals, were influenced by smells, as I learnt later. Spelling meant smelling and decimals were smells, which cut the whole number, her mother's body, into ten parts. The use of musculature was inhibited too, because movement was felt by her to lead to the most severe attacks on her mother's body. She was slow in starting to walk. The bulk of the oral lavatory contents had to be added to the anal and urethral one and eliminated through the cloaca. I learnt later in the analysis that she was constipated until she started menstruating, that is, until her third lavatory hole, her vagina, was opened to her for evacuation as well. In this amphimixis (Ferenczi [1924]) the anxieties related to every organ and function were condensed. The restricted elimination of the bad contents at all levels influenced the introduction of good objects and substances at all levels. She felt herself small. Her introjection was inhibited in eating, sublimations, and in intercourse.

In passing I would like to mention a hypothesis concerning wind, which has occurred to me in the analysis of this patient – supported by two other cases I am treating. The significance of flatus, its hidden omnipotent nature pervading the whole field of bodily and mental expressions, is a fact well known in psychoanalytic literature since Jones [1912]. The importance of breathing, wind and smells to my patient and the observation of infants from their first day at the breast led me to assume that at the beginning of breast feeding the infant in many cases cannot enjoy the milk or the breast because it has to adapt its breathing to the drinking, it has to find a satisfactory rhythm. Dr Balint [1948] investigated this. The ideal object at this stage is felt to be the nipple that protects the infant from suffocation and from cutting the breast with aggressive breathing and wind. The aggressive breathing and the wind are later merged with the flatus in the anal elimination, and add to the flatus the most primitive omnipotent qualities. Normally a gratifying feeding and a gratifying breast are soon established by the newly born infant. In my patient this does not seem to have been the case. From the beginning there was an interaction between her impulses – oral vampire and cutting wind, and the handling by the grossly depressed mother who lived in fear that her husband would be called up. A fixation on this level influenced her mode of introjection and projection of objects at later levels and her sexual development, as I hope to substantiate more fully in further material. It is interesting in this context that among her widespread phobic formations and fears none concerned teeth. I naturally anticipated finding indications of fear of biting, cutting by gums and teeth, but as far as I could see, in my patient the fear of attacking and cutting her mother's breast was specifically related to wind and screams.[7] The importance of early screaming was described by Nina Searl [1933]. I came to the conclusion that the patient's anxieties from the first day or days at the breast, about cutting and poisoning the breast by wind – flatus – deeply inhibited her biting impulse.[8] In phantasy her vampire mouth only sucked the blood out of the nipple.

Gradual improvement followed and new conflicts and fears emerged. This was also expressed in a change of dream contents, which now became stealing dreams. In the last lavatory dream the progress was expressed in a more adult and realistic conception in the genital part of the dream. Instead of dancing with the prince it was represented through a couple who had children and who liked their job, intercourse. The conflict was expressed in the next part in which she was sitting on a lavatory and a penis four times the normal size was hanging between her legs. The word penis, used for the first time by the patient in this dream,[9] was introduced in the lavatory, hanging from her lavatory vagina. The move from anal to genital ushered in the oedipal conflict on this level, her penis envy and exhibitionistic impulses. Her defence was a degradation of intercourse making it into lavatory intercourse. In connection with this dream the patient told me that her parents expected her to be a boy.

In this period her fears of intercourse and childbirth were brought to analysis and expressed through stealing dreams. The penis envy provides a link to the stealing. As a child she stole an engine from her cousin. She did not think she stole it because her uncle said: 'Wouldn't you like it'. She thought he meant her to have it. But in fear of her mother she gave it away. The theft was never discovered and it haunted her all her life.

The first stealing dream came after a weekend. She started by telling me she had felt so well on Saturday and spontaneously suggested to her husband a walk for the first time since her breakdown. On the walk they contemplated building a bungalow. But on Sunday she couldn't leave the house. A fragment of the dream is that she bought a silver entrée dish at a sale. Her mother, sister and mother-in-law were with her. Before she left one of them put a silver spoon in her bag. The patient cried out, 'Take it out, people might think I have stolen it'. The weekend and the dream repeated the weekend she got married. She set out full of hopes and felt humiliated and exposed in intercourse as in the dream. The guilt over having frustrated the sexual life of her mother and mother figures, sister and mother-in-law prevented her from having intercourse. Reparation she felt was not possible because her husband's penis would have to gratify in intercourse not only herself but [also] the three mother figures inside her. For this she would need the four times sized penis from her lavatory dreams. It made the penis into the persecuting object for which she felt too small and was afraid that it would shatter her. Depression made her regress[10] into persecution and the self-reproaches changed into accusations against her mother. She accused her treacherous mother that she frustrated her sexual life from birth. It was her mother who stole her penis, because her father meant her to be born with the silver spoon penis, as the uncle meant her to have the engine. And so throughout her life, culminating in not letting her have her husband's penis. She could not have intercourse because her husband's penis stood for her mother's penis, with which she [mother] would force herself in and scoop her out. The patient utilised this penis envy as a defence against her guilt about frustrating the parents' intercourse. There was ample material to confirm this.

Another symptom appeared at this time, the fear of reading. It started with looking into a *Woman's Own* belonging to her landlady whilst she was out. She couldn't read a book or even a timetable because she was afraid she would not be able to get back to her normal self.

The next dream dealt with her fears of having a baby. She dreamt it was Wednesday early closing and she expected a couple for a meal. She pulled out a stick of rhubarb from her landlady's garden to go with an egg pudding.

She was in a large brick kitchen, not her own. An uninvited woman was with her. The patient broke many eggs, because they were smelly and mixed with blood, although they were her rationed M[inistry of] F[ood] eggs. In the garden she pulled out many thin sticks of rhubarb before she found a short[11] thick one. She did not know where to hide all the leaves. She had already filled up the dustbin. She woke in fear. Some of her associations were to the eggs mixed with blood, a mad thought about dead-born babies, miscarriages, and this was mixed up in her mind with menstruation. It reminded her of the talks between her mother and Mrs P about childbirth which used to make her sick when she was a child. Mrs P had many miscarriages. Her youngest was prematurely born but grew up into a healthy married woman with a baby.

It emerged from the analysis of the dream that the pudding stood for her baby with which she wanted to revive her parents whose life had an early closing. But added to the guilt over the stolen rhubarb penis was her greater guilt over raiding and destroying her mother's body. She broke into her mother's womb, the kitchen, and destroyed there the potential fertility of the parental genitals, the eggs and the rhubarb, mixed them up with faeces, and left her mother a full-up dust-bin, lavatory. No child was born after her. She took [and] ate the fresh fertilised eggs and the thick rhubarb, the erect penis. She could neither use them inside her to make the baby nor hide the leaves [or] left-overs with which she was full. The uninvited woman in her kitchen standing for the revengeful and triumphing mother inside her was watching her breaking her eggs and mixing them with blood and faeces. She felt fear but not guilt. This had been dealt with in the familiar manner. She accused her mother, the Ministry of Food, that she rationed her between feeds instead of feeding her non-stop and closed, weaned her too early. Her mother was responsible that she confused genital and procreative processes with excretory ones and for her mad thoughts about them, because she never explained it to her. Therefore she can't have a baby, it would make her mad.

There is some hope however in this dream. She is in the role of the premature baby whom I, standing for Mrs P the expert on child rearing, will bring up into a healthy married woman with a baby. She is also in the role of her mother being able to have talks with Mrs P, me, the expert on conception, pregnancy and childbirth.

The patient was gradually able to open up and I got from her the history of her marital sexual relationships. She told me they continued the attempts at intercourse about once a month. Her husband tried to penetrate but she tensed up and he had an ejaculation. At the beginning of every attempt she was excited but it passed quickly and she was bored. Her contempt for and hate of her husband came out more into the open. She accused him of being impotent, inexperienced, bored and causing all her fears of intercourse because had he put more effort in at their first intercourse she would not have become so ill, and so on, a repetition of her accusations against her mother. After these persecutory anxieties had been worked through to some extent conscious wishes for intercourse came up. She would have liked to discuss it with him and knew that he waited for an opportunity. There were dreams in which she brought him to me, I should talk to him. After a weekend dream to which she had difficulties to associate, she said: 'There isn't anything, I don't want to think'. When I pointed out that she repeated her intercourse situation with me, the dream being the genital which she exposed to me and I was to put all my effort into it whilst she tensed up, she said they had had a sort of intercourse on Friday. She let him penetrate further than ever before but he couldn't get right up, she tensed up again. She realised that intercourse was normal, not mad as she had thought pre viously but she still had fears. She was afraid that the penis would get stuck in her. For the first time after their nine years of marriage she was able to discuss it with her husband and discovered that he had thought that she did not want intercourse. She herself had believed that he did not want intercourse and was bored by it.[12]

The patient's fear of intercourse was intensified by her fears relating to having a baby. Through the equation penis baby, the intercourse felt to her to be pregnancy and childbirth all at once. The central fear of intercourse was the fear that her mother's penis, represented by her husband's penis, would retaliate in her intercourse for all the attacks she felt she made on her mother's breast and body. It would cling to her and get stuck in her vagina. It would eat up the inside of her womb and make her into a womb lavatory filled with disintegrated bits of the self. In her phantasy her mother's penis represented the penis that her father left to her mother to give to her, as symbolised by the silver spoon penis.[13] Conversely, she was afraid that her vagina was the vampire mouth that would trap and suck out the protecting penis and ingest it in her womb into miscarriages, dead babies, or mentally and physically damaged babies. She felt that her womb contained disintegrated bits of her mother's body, parental genitals and . . . the self. These she split off and displaced into her head. She felt them as mad thoughts racing through her head, confusing her [and] threatening her with madness.

To escape from the dangerous internal claustra and their contents she projected them outside. The breast claustrum, as I have described, she projected into the garment and into the running water. The inside of the body, the womb claustrum which contained the parental genitals in intercourse she projected into theatres, cinemas, etc. The uterus as a claustrum was described by Jones [1912] and Ferenczi [1922]. The head claustrum with the mad thoughts in it she projected into books and any reading matter. The fears, symptoms and inhibitions were related to the organs and substances with which she felt she attacked her mother's breast and body:

1   The fear of losing her voice, her sight, her mind, [and] the power of her legs. They stand also for stolen penises with which she felt she forced herself into her mother's body and would be trapped and castrated.
2   The symptoms of choking and not being able to swallow, sore throats, heaving, colics and constipation are the concomitants of the process of ingestion of the raided and retaliating contents and parts of her mother's body. Here belong the inhibitions in food with regard to eggs, fish and offal, and the intellectual inhibitions.

My conclusion is that the central phobia of my patient is the phobia of sexual intercourse, the traumatic situation as Freud discovered in which internal and external dangers converge. The danger as my patient felt it was the death of the internal and external object and the disintegration of the self. Her main defence against it was a defence of immobility, of suspension. She managed neither to consummate her marriage nor to break it off. This state of suspension she had been able to maintain since childhood with the help of her claustrophobic symptoms and inhibitions and with the help of protecting objects. The marriage through intercourse threatened a breakdown of these defences. She kept the first year of her marriage going by sore throats. The fear of throwing herself from the window brought her to ana lysis. The extensive use of the defences I mentioned. . . [was] a barrage against guilt and depression, which the patient was not able to work through in her life. External factors contributed to this at every crucial point in her development.

1   Her first psychological environment was a depressed mother who lived in fear that her husband would be called up.
2   At the age of one, still under the sway of the weaning and at the height of the anal stage, there was no father to turn to – on the contrary she felt she

had to be her mother's companion and be concerned for the ill and depressed mother.

3   At the age of four and a half, at her father's return, a flaring up of the oedipal conflict in frustration and hate leading to a tie with a hated mother figure, her sister, throughout latency.

4   At adolescence her father's death and a renewed tie to her mother.

5   At marriage the death of her mother.

The interaction of internal and external factors resulted in a personality structure consisting of: (a) a cruelly torturing superego, [partially constituted by] the internalised father who died prematurely, and a buried alive mother; (b) a crippled genital libido; and (c) an infantile ego with little reality sense, unable to cope with the demands made upon it.

I have tried to show in this paper that the earliest anxieties relating to the introjection of the breast influenced all later introjections and contributed to my patient's fear of intercourse. The attacks on her mother's body – breast, womb and head – with oral, anal cutting impulses, made it into a body containing three cavities: the breast, the womb, [and] the head claustra. These were emptied of the good contents and filled with bad ones. Through introjective and projective processes they became her internal and external claustra. Through amphimixis all the anxieties relating to the mouth were condensed in her vagina cloaca. The equation penis breast baby made the penis into the most persecuting object.

These anxieties influenced the character of the ideal object. The object and its function were split. The ideal object was a small part of the breast, the nipple, and a corresponding small part of the penis. Their function was not to gratify but to protect from fear by non-penetration – immobility. Penetrating intercourse meant the loss of the protecting object in the phobic situation.

In conclusion, I will mention briefly the results of the analysis so far. Through the diminution of persecutory anxieties towards mother figures, the patient was able to enjoy the relationships with her two women friends by whom previously she felt victimised and humiliated. She is more tolerant of her husband, can allow him the male role in external affairs and feels relieved by it, can show him affection and tries to please him. She is aware of the change in her personality and in her relationships with people. This gives her increased hope that she will be able to enjoy sexual intercourse. Most of her other symptoms have disappeared.

Acknowledgements

The original of the present paper is preserved among the W.C.M. Scott papers at the National Archives of Canada, Ottawa, under reference MG31, 57.19. Acknowledgement is here made to them and particularly their Archivist, Larry McNally, for facilitating access to the paper, and to Miss Betty Joseph, Esther Bick's executor, for permission to publish it here. Recently two further copies of this paper have come to light, in the libraries of the Institute of Psychoanalysis and the Tavistock Clinic in London.

Notes

1 Originally published in the *British Journal of Psychotherapy,* Vol. 18 (1), 2001.
2 Esther Bick was a member of the British Psychoanalytical Society, qualified in both adult and child analysis and, along with John Bowlby, founded the Tavistock Clinic's child psychotherapy training. This paper has been edited by Roger Willoughby. Address for correspondence: 8 Castle Hill Avenue, Folkestone, Kent, CT20 2QT; email: roger@willoughbywarren.com.
3 In his comments on Bick's paper, Winnicott was particularly critical of her use of 'splitting' as a concept, which he suggested reflected a failure to adequately distinguish between the radical splitting in schizophrenia and dissociation that occurs within more neurotic personalities, a confusion that he thought was characteristic of the Kleinian group. See *The Spontaneous Gesture*: *Selected Letters of D.W. Winnicott*, edited by F.R. Rodman, Cambridge, MA: Harvard, 1987, pp. 51–52.
4 This phrase, 'regress from depression', was a manuscript change, written in lieu of the words 'turn guilt'. Winnicott later criticized Bick's use of this phrase, writing that it 'means nothing at all as it stands . . . I suppose you are referring to Melanie Klein's concept of a paranoid position in emotional development, which I consider one of her less well worked out theories'; see Rodman, op. cit. p. 51.
5 Bertram Lewin had begun to popularize this term, first using it in his 1952 paper 'Phobic symptoms and dream interpretation', *Psychoanal. Q.*, 21: 295–322.
6 Bick modified the original text here, which had read 'These feel to her to be. . .'
7 Originally this sentence began with 'I was naturally inclined to find indications of fear of biting, cutting by gums and teeth, but I came to be convinced so far that in my patient. . .' Bick's replacement text tempered the overall tone.
8 This sentence and the next were later additions penned into the typescript.
9 The phrase 'in this dream' was a later manuscript addition.
10 This phrase, penned in later, replaced 'The guilt was turned. . .' Winnicott's comments (see note 2) apply here also.
11 This word was a later addition.
12 This sentence was added later by hand.
13 This sentence was added later by hand.

References

Balint, M. (1948). Individual Differences of Behaviour in Early Infancy and an Objective Method for Recording Them. *Journal of Genetic Psychology*, *73*:57–117.
Bick, E. (1968). The Experience of the Skin in Early Object-Relations. *International Journal of Psychoanalysis*, 49:484–486.
Bick, E. (1986). Further Considerations on the Function of the Skin in Early Object Relations: Findings from Infant Observation Integrated into Child and Adult Analysis. *British Journal of Psychotherapy*, 2:292–299.
Bion, W.R. (1962). *Learning from Experience*. Heinemann.
Deutsch, H. (1929). The Genesis of Agoraphobia. *International Journal of Psychoanalysis*, *10*:51–69.
Fenichel, O. (1944). Remarks on the Common Phobias. *Psychoanalytic Quarterly, 13*:313–326.

Ferenczi, S. (1922). Bridge Symbolism and the Don Juan Legend (1994 Edition). In *Further Contributions to the Theory and Technique of Psychoanalysis* (pp. 356–358). Karnac.

Ferenczi, S. (1924). *Thalassa: A Theory of Genitality* (1989 Edition). Karnac.

Freud, S. (1926). Inhibitions, Symptoms and Anxiety. In *SE* (Vol. 20). Hogarth Press.

Gillespie, W.H. (1953). Extra-sensory Elements in Dream Interpretation. In *Psychoanalysis and the Occult*. International Universities Press.

Jones, E. (1912). *Papers on Psycho-Analysis* (1923 Edition, 3rd edition). W.M. Wood.

Klein, M. (1932). *The Psychoanalysis of Children* (1980 Edition). Hogarth Press.

Klein, M. (1935). A Contribution to the Psychogenesis of Manic-Depressive States. *International Journal of Psychoanalysis*, *16*:145–174.

Klein, M. (1940). Mourning and Its Relation to Manic-Depressive States. *International Journal of Psychoanalysis*, *21*:125–153.

Klein, M. (1945). The Oedipus Complex in the Light of Early Anxieties (1985 Edition). In *Love, Guilt and Reparation and Other Works, 1921–1945* (pp. 370–419). Hogarth Press.

Klein, M. (1946). Notes on Some Schizoid Mechanisms (1984 Edition). In *Envy and Gratitude and Other Works, 1946–1963* (pp. 1–24). Hogarth Press.

Lewin, B.D. (1933). The Body as Phallus. *Psychoanalytic Quarterly*, *2*:24–47.

Lewin, B.D. (1935). Claustrophobia. *Psychoanalytic Quarterly*, *4*:227–233.

Lewin, B.D. (1952). Phobic Symptoms and Dream Interpretation. *Psychoanalytic Quarterly*, *21*:295–322.

Meltzer, D. (1967). The Psycho-Analytical Process. *The Psycho-analytical Process*, *138*:1–109.

Oberndorf, C. (1929). Submucous Resection as a Castration Symbol. *International Journal of Psychoanalysis*, *10*:228–241.

Rey, J.H. (1988). That Which Patients Bring to Analysis. *International Journal of Psychoanalysis*, *69*:457–470.

Searl, N.M. (1933). The Psychology of Screaming. *International Journal of Psychoanalysis*, *14*:193–205.

Winnicott, D. (1963). Dependence in Infant Care, in Child Care, and in the Psycho-Analytic Setting. *International Journal of Psychoanalysis*, *44*:339–344.

Winnicott, D. (1974). Fear of Breakdown. *International Review of Psychoanalysis*, *1*:103.

Chapter 5

The Relation of Anal Masturbation to Projective Identification[1]

Donald Meltzer[2]

SUMMARY

Meltzer argues that anal masturbation is more commonplace than previously recognized and results in a character constellation of 'pseudo-maturity' and anal eroticism. The narcissistic valuation of faeces causes confusion in the anal zones: anus-vagina and penis-faeces. He links the obsessional and perverse character traits of anal masturbation, projective identification, and pseudo-maturity as a defence against dependency. In 1935 (Chapter 3), Weiss describes a similar concept of pseudo-development as a defensive structure against dependency.

Pseudo-maturity occurs during the feeding situation, when the nursling, in phantasy, intrusively projects himself into the mother's breasts, then into her bottom when she turns away. The baby then equates the mother's buttocks with her breasts and her bottom with his own bottom. This results in an idealization of the rectum as a source of food and delusional projective identification with the internal mother that erases the differentiation between child and adult regarding capacities and prerogatives.

The confusion of which body part belongs to whom causes the baby to live an idealized phantasy existence inside the mother's bottom (or anal claustrum). This experience is reminiscent of Henri Rey's (1994, p. 7) famous quote: 'What part of the subject, situated where in space and time, is doing what to what part of the object, situated where in space and time and with what motivations and with what consequences for the subject and object?'

The internal combined parental couple is seen in phantasy as viciously attacking one another. In childhood, the character crust of intolerance and criticism of others is vulnerable to breaking down, resulting in tantrums, cruelty, lying, and suicide. Hypochondriacal and claustrophobic anxieties are a consequence of this narcissistic character structure. As the Oedipus complex is bypassed, this leaves both the child and adult vulnerable to 'pseudo-adjustment' and feelings of fraudulence.

Analysis with this type of character perversion is vulnerable to breaking down, as the patient is pseudo-cooperative and seductive, enslaving the analyst to join the idealization of pseudo-maturity by soliciting praise, approval, and admiration

DOI: 10.4324/9781003200284-5

from the analyst while simultaneously attacking him. Meltzer states that progress can still be accomplished in spite of the acting-out behavior if the analyst is able to elucidate the cryptic masturbation and succeed in dream analysis.

Meltzer's later writing agrees with Mason's conclusions of claustrophobia as a defence against psychosis and a super-ego that is suffocating (Mason, Chapter 6). Meltzer's concept of the gang is related to Rosenfeld's narcissistic object relations and to Steiner's psychic retreats (Chapter 8). Meltzer's later concepts of toilet breast and compartmentalization of geographic locations were influenced by his supervisor and collaborator Esther Bick (Chapter 4).

TEXT

Introduction

When attempting to relate some character traits of the 'Wolf Man' to his intestinal symptoms, Freud (1918) was forced to the conclusion that an anal theory of femininity and an 'identification' with his mother's menorrhagia had antedated the patient's castration theory of femininity. Until Melanie Klein's establishment of the concept of 'projective identification' it was assumed that such a process would have been due solely to introjection. In her original description (1957 [1946], p. 300) of projective identification, Klein linked it very closely to anal processes but nowhere else in her written work has this connexion been made more explicit.

Furthermore, the contribution made by anality to character formation, as studied by Freud (1908, 1917), Abraham (1921), Jones (1913, 1918), Heimann (1962), and others, has always been stated in terms of the outcome in character structure of the so-called 'sublimation' of anal fantasies, in which the emphasis has rested on the narcissistic over-evaluation of the faeces on the one hand and the object-relationship consequences of the toilet-training struggle on the other. The present paper intends to demonstrate the contribution to character formation made by the combination of all three factors working in complex relation to one another, namely narcissistic evaluation of the faeces, the confusions surrounding the anal zone (especially anus-vagina and penis-faeces confusions) and the identification aspect of anal habits and fantasies based on projective identification. In studying this problem in the analytic process, in close collaboration with several colleagues, I have been forced also to the recognition that masturbation of the anus is a far more widespread habit than the analytic literature to date would imply. Freud (1905, p. 187); (1917, p. 131) recognized its existence in children who employ both fingers and the faecal mass as the masturbatory object. However, Spitz's (1949) study of faecal play and his conclusions, based on observational and not analytic data, have promulgated an implication of severe pathology not substantiated by our own work.

For the sake of presentation, and partly to accord with the Congress theme of the Obsessional States, this paper is also focused on the character constellation of 'pseudo-maturity' which we find to be intimately related to anal erotism, a finding by no means at variance with the descriptions by Winnicott (1965) and by Deutsch (1942) of what they have called the 'false self' and the 'as if' personality type respectively. The relation of 'pseudo-maturity' to obsessional states will be demonstrated and shown to assume an oscillatory system at a certain stage of the analytic process, throwing some light on the background of obsessional character in a manner similar to the description of the cyclothymic background of obsessional neurosis given in my earlier (1963) paper. Clinical material and theoretical discussion will bind together the three concepts: anal masturbation, projective identification, pseudo-maturity.

The Characerology

Inadequate splitting-and-idealization (Klein 1957), operative particularly after weaning, in relation to demands for cleanliness and aggravated by the expectation or arrival of younger siblings, contributes to a strong trend to idealize the Rectum and its faecal contents. But this idealization is largely based on a confusion of identity due to the operation of projective identification, whereby the baby's bottom and that of the mother are confused one with the other, and both are equated with the mother's breasts.

As we reconstruct the scene from the analytic situation a typical sequence would appear as follows: after a feed, when placed in the cot, as mother walks away, the baby, hostilely equating mother's breasts with her buttocks, begins to explore its own bottom, idealizing its roundness and smoothness and eventually penetrating the anus to reach the retained, withheld faeces. In this process of penetration, a fantasy of secret intrusion into mother's anus (Abraham 1921, p. 389) to rob her takes shape, whereby the baby's rectal contents become confused with mother's idealized faeces, felt to be withheld by her to feed daddy and the inside-babies.

The consequence of this is twofold, namely an idealization of the rectum as a source of food and the projective (delusional) identification with the internal mother which erases the differentiation between child and adult as regards capacities and prerogatives. The urine and flatus may also come in for their share of idealization.

In the excited and confused state which results from the anal masturbation, a bimanual masturbation of genital (phallus or clitoris) and anus (confused with vagina) tends to ensue, producing a sado-masochistic perverse coital fantasy in which the internal parental couple do great harm to one another. The projective identification with both internal figures which accompanies this bimanual masturbation harms the internal objects both by the violence of intrusion into them and by the sadistic nature of the intercourse it produces between them. Hypochondria as well as claustrophobic anxieties are thus an invariable consequence to some degree.

In childhood this situation encourages a pre-oedipal (ages 2–3) crystallization of character manifest by docility, helpfulness, preference for adult companionship, aloofness or bossiness with other children, intolerance of criticism, and high verbal capacity. When this characterological crust is broken momentarily by frustration or anxiety, outcrops of hair-raising virulence are laid bare – tantrums, faecal smearing, suicidal attempts, vicious assaults on other children, lying to strangers about parental maltreatment, cruelty to animals, etc.

This structure by-passes the Oedipus complex and seems to equip a child reasonably well superficially for academic and social life and may carry through into adulthood relatively unruffled even by the adolescent upheaval. But the 'pseudo' nature of the adjustment is apparent in adult life even where the perverse tendencies have not led to obviously aberrant sexual activities. The feeling of fraudulence as an adult person, the sexual impotence or pseudo-potency (excited by secret perverse fantasies), the inner loneliness and the basic confusion between good and bad, all create a life of tension and lack of satisfaction, bolstered, or rather compensated, only by the smugness and snobbery which are an inevitable accompaniment of the massive projective identification.

Where this organization is less dominant and pervasive, or during analysis when it begins to give way to the therapeutic process, it stands in an oscillatory relation to an obsessional organization. There the internal objects are not penetrated, but are rather omnipotently controlled and separated on a less part-object level of relationship, as the focal difficulties have moved from separation anxieties toward the previously by-passed oedipal conflicts.

The delusional identification with the mother due to projective identification and the confusion between anus and vagina together produce frigidity and a sense of fraudulent femininity in women. In men these dynamics produce either homosexual activities or more frequently an intense dread of becoming homosexual (since the heightened femininity is not distinguished from passive anal homosexuality). Or conversely the secondary projective identification with the father's penis (in the ensuing bimanual masturbation) may produce a leading phallic quality in either male or female patients especially where omnipotent (manic) reparativeness has been mobilized as a defence against the severe underlying depression present in all such cases.

The Nature of the Transference

When this configuration of massive projective identification with the internal objects, usually on a part-object level as breast or penis, is active the cooperation of an adult sort in the analytic process is replaced by a pseudocooperation or 'helpfulness' to the analyst. This acting out shows itself in a somewhat slavish demeanour, a desire to convince, to demonstrate, to assist, or to relieve the analyst of his burdens. Material is therefore often of a predigested variety, sometimes given in 'headline' fashion or as superficial interpretations of mental states. All sense of the patient's wishing to elicit interpretation is absent, replaced by an evident desire for praise, approval, admiration, or even gratitude from the analyst. When these are not forthcoming, the analyst's activities are often felt to evince lack of understanding, envious attacks on the patient's capacities, mere surliness, or frank sadism. This latter reception of interpretation can quickly lead to erotization and cause the interpretation to be experienced as a sexual assault.

Whether the patient is producing dreams, associations, or a factual account of his daily activities, the acting out aspect is so dominant that the interpretation of content is relatively useless unless coupled with a clear demonstration of the nature and basis of the behaviour. This of course results in sullenness of the nothing-I-ever-do-pleases-you variety. But by the painstaking demonstration of the acting out, by consistent elucidation of the cryptic masturbation, and finally through dream analysis, progress can usually be made.

Acting out of the infantile projective identification with internal figures is such a prominent part of the character that its continual demonstration as a contaminant in the patient's adult life must be undertaken. Even in the face of intense opposition this scrutiny must also include areas of the greatest pride, success, and apparent satisfaction such as work, 'creative' activities, relations to children, siblings, or continued solicitous helpfulness to aging parents. The significance of clothing for the women, cars for the men, and money-in-the-bank for all must be investigated, for they are sure to be found loaded with irrational significance. So skilled is the counterfeiting of maturity in thought, attitude, communication, and action that only the dreams make possible this teasing apart of infantile 'pseudo-mature' items from the adult pattern of life.

The Dreams

It is worth mentioning here that sensitivity to the anal masturbatory aspects of the adult patient's dreams is immeasurably increased by experience with child patients and psychotics. Much of what appears below derives its conviction from such sources:

a   Idealization of the faeces as food – dreams of scavenging and finding are in this category: finding apples among the autumn leaves, food in the empty larder, reaching into places the inside of which cannot be visualized, or underneath structures. Fishing and hunting may also come into this category, though not generally; but gardening, shopping, and stealing of food do, especially if the place is represented as dark, dirty, cheap or foreign.

b   Idealization of the rectum – dreams in which the rectum is represented as a retreat or refuge generally show it as an eating place (restaurant or café, kitchen or dining room) but with qualities which announce its significance. It may be dirty, dark, smelly, cheap, crowded, smoky, below ground level, noisy, run by foreigners, in a foreign city. The food may be unappetizing, unhygienic, unhealthy, fattening, overcooked, homogeneous (custards, puddings, etc.), or catering to infantile greed in quantity or sweetness. Where rectum and breast are confused such configuration as outdoor cafés or market places with the above characteristics may appear.

c   Idealization of the toilet situation (Abraham 1920, p. 318) – this often appears
     in dreams as sitting in lofty or exciting places, often looking down at water
     (lakes, canyons, streams) or sitting in places where food is being prepared, or
     in a position of importance ('Last Supper' dreams) or where people behind
     the dreamer are waiting for food, payment, services, or information (conduct-
     ing an orchestra, serving at an altar).
d   Representation of the anally masturbating fingers – these appear in dreams
     represented as parts of the body, people, animals, tools or machines, either
     singly or in groups of four or five, with qualities of faecal contamination vari-
     ously represented or denied, such as negroes, men in brown helmets, soiled
     or shiny garden tools, white gloves, people dressed in black, earth-moving
     tractors, dirty children, worms, rusty nails, etc.
e   Dreams showing the process of intrusion into the anus of the object (Abra-
     ham 1921, p. 389) – most frequently seen as entering a building or a vehicle,
     either furtively, by a back entrance, the door has wet paint, the entrance is
     very narrow, protective clothing must be worn, it is underground, underwater,
     in a foreign country or closed to the public, etc.
f   Idealization of the rectum as a source of pseudo-analysis – this is frequent
     and may appear as secondhand bookshops, piles of old newspapers, filing
     cabinets, public libraries – one patient before an examination dreamed that he
     fished in the Fleet Street sewer and caught an encyclopaedia.

Clinical Material

I have chosen the following material to show the complexity of the connexions to
orality and genitality which infuse the anal masturbatory situation and its attendant projective identification with such defensive power.

Three years of analytic work with a late adolescent young man had begun to press
toward the dependent relationship to the breast which his history suggested would
be extremely disturbed, for he had been a poor feeder, a complaining baby, and a
tyrannical child in his dependence on his mother. We knew something of his capacity for scathing mockery and of a terrible way of laughing contemptuously, but this
had seldom been unleashed in the consulting room, where his behaviour tended to
be superficially cooperative, 'churning out fantasies', as he called it, all with an air
of insincerity which made even the simplest account of a daily happening sound like
confabulation. This we had already understood as 'pretending to be insincere' but
indistinguishable to himself from 'pretending to pretend to be insincere', all of which
related to a deeply fixed paranoid feeling of being overheard by a hidden persecutor.

He dreamed that he was among friends and seemed once again, as in school
days, to be the head boy. As they came over the *brow* of a hill, he saw a man,
whom he knew to be a murderer, among some gravestones, just wandering about.

Reassuring his friends that he knew how to handle the man, he approached him
with an aide and, pretending to be friendly, led him down to the *bottom*, hoping
to extract a confession.

ASSOCIATIONS – his tongue seems to be exploring the back of his teeth which feel old and cracked. That makes him think of putting on some slippers like the ones his father used to have. INTERPRETATION – that his teeth are represented by the gravestones and his tongue as the murderer among his victims. His device in the dream is to rid his mouth of these dangerous qualities and transform them into slippery fingers which can be led down to his bottom, where the victims can be identified in his faeces. But by this device his finger-in-his-bottom becomes confused with father's penis-in-mother's-vagina, an important source of the Nazi-daddy-who-kills-mummy's-Jewish-babies whom we know so well from earlier work. ASSOCIATIONS – he feels as if a circular saw were cutting his thigh (reference to surgery for hernia in puberty). He imagines himself with his back to double doors and the analyst outside trying to pull them open (projection of the buttock-spreading onto the analyst-surgeon-daddy). ASSOCIATIONS – an ornately carved gilt picture frame (the analyst's interpretation is an ornate picture intended to frame him by revealing his guilt), the Mafia – the black hand. A boat going through a canal which is shaped to fit its keel-less hull (the Mafia-fascist daddy getting the big black penis-finger into his anal canal, reassuring him in an Italian accent: 'No keel!').

These associations are typical of the punning which characterizes the compulsive anal masturbatory fantasies.

Four weeks later, approaching the Christmas holiday, in a state of mounting resentment and increasing difficulty at work due to acting out, he came fifteen minutes late and tracked mud from an unpaved road (a shortcut from the underground station to the consulting room) into my room. Only once before had he done this.

ASSOCIATIONS – he had rubbishy dreams over the week-end and feels reluctant to impose them on the analyst. INTERPRETATION – this conscious wish to spare is contrasted by an unconscious wish to dirty the analyst inside and out with his faeces, a bit of which has been acted out by tracking the dirt into the room. Patient looked with surprise at the floor, and apologised. ASSOCIATIONS – On Saturday night he dreamed he was tossing and turning in pain due to a dislocated finger (shows uninjured left index finger). INTERPRETATION – link with the gravestone dream. The week-end distress felt as due to the removal of his murderer-finger (Mafia) from its accustomed location. ASSOCIATIONS – but then he seemed at school, idle and bored. He wandered into the men's lavatory, where there seemed to be a nice big clean bathtub. He decided to have a bath, but then it changed to a small, filthy station toilet with pornographic writing and pictures on the wall, just opposite the basement of a big department store. He couldn't decide what to do, because the staff of the store kept watching him suspiciously. He kept going in and out of the lavatory, until finally he entered the store to steal something.

This dream shows with unusual clarity the way in which the current separation situation (the dislocated finger at the boring week-end) leads to a sequence of infantile events, first wetting himself (the bath) with warm urine, then exploring his anus (the filthy toilet), becoming more and more sexually aroused (the pornography) and preoccupied with projective identification fantasies about the bottom of mother's body (the toilet-rectum across from the department-store-vagina with the watchful staff-penis) and his wish to rob her.

Sunday night's dream, approaching with some anxiety the Monday session, reveals the continuation of the infantile state, now a baby with soiled nappy, bottom, and cot. In the dream he wanted to change his clothes for a party he and friends were giving at his flat, but already every room was filled with guests, laughing, drinking and smoking (his soiled cot and nappy). But then he was in the park and felt happy among the greenery, even though he had on nothing but an undershirt (the baby has kicked off its nappy and idealizes its soiled bottom and cot). He finds a football to kick and soon others have joined him in the game (playing with his faeces).

This latter state, self-idealization through athletics, had appeared literally in hundreds of dreams in the first two years of his analysis. Here we see in detail its derivation. It is worth mentioning that this patient had suffered from a chronic, but non-ulcerative diarrhoea since early childhood which had only abated some eight months earlier in the analysis.

The Cryptic Anal Masturbation

Reconstruction from the transference indicates that anal masturbation becomes cryptic very early in childhood and tends to remain both unnoticed and unrecognized in its significance thereafter, except when frank perversions declare themselves in adolescence or later. I have referred to it as 'cryptic' to emphasise here the unconscious skill with which it is hidden from scrutiny.

The most common form (see Freud, and Abraham) utilizes the faecal mass itself as the masturbatory stimulant. Either its retention, slow expulsion, rhythmic partial expulsion and retraction, or the rapid, forced, and painful expulsion are accompanied by the unconscious fantasies which alter the ego state. This change in mental state can be noted in child patients when they return from defaecating during sessions. The habit of reading on the toilet, special methods of cleansing the anus, special concern about leaving a bad smell, anxiety about faecal stain on underclothing, habitually dirty finger nails, surreptitious smelling of fingers, etc. all are tentative indicators of cryptic anal masturbation. But it can skilfully be hidden far afield from the act of defaecation: in bathing habits, the wearing of constrictive undergarments, in cycling, horseback riding or other activities which stimulate the buttocks. Most difficult perhaps of all to locate is the sequestration of anal masturbation in the genital sexual relation, which is invariably the case to some extent while anus and vagina are still confused with one another. On the other hand, like Poe's 'Purloined Letter', it may be flamboyantly in view, as in constipation with enemata, suppositories for recurrent fissure *in ano*, etc. but its significance denied.

While it is not part of my technique to comment on a patient's behaviour on the couch nor to ask for associations to it, scrutiny of the patterns of posture and movement and linking them with dream material does sometimes permit a fruit-ful interpretation of the behaviour. By this means the series of modifications of the anal masturbation can be revealed and a more successful search for the actual anal stimulation instituted. For instance, a patient who often kept both hands in his pockets recognized through a dream that this was accompanied at times by pulling at a loose thread. This led to the realization that he had a habit of manually teasing apart peri-anal hairs prior to defaecation lest they spoil the shape of his emerging faecal mass.

The Analytic Process

The early years of analysis in such cases involve primarily the resolution of the self-idealization and spurious independence, through the establishment of the capacity in the transference to utilize the analytic breast for projective relief (the toilet-breast). The relief of confusional states (Klein 1957) takes the forefront, especially those confusions of identity and therefore about time and the adult-child differ-ential which characterize massive projective identification. It is only after several years, when the attachment to the feeding breast is developing and the intolerance to separations is rhythmically being invoked at week-ends and holidays, that these processes can be accurately and fruitfully investigated. It seems certain that, unless the cryptic anal masturbation can be discovered and its insidious production of aberrant ego states scotched at source, further progress is seriously impeded.

This brings us to a most important point in our exposition, for I would suggest from my experience that the dynamic here described is often of such a subtle struc-ture, the pressure on the analyst to join in the idealization of the pseudo-maturity so great, and the underlying threats of psychosis and suicide so covertly com-municated that many of the 'successful' analyses which break down months or years after termination may fall into this category. It is necessary therefore also to stress that the countertransference position is extremely difficult and in every way repeats the dilemma of the parents, who found themselves with a 'model' child, so long as they abstained from being distinctly parental, either in the form of author-ity, teaching, or opposition to the relatively modest claims for privileges beyond those to which the child's age and accomplishments could reasonably entitle it.

This seductiveness must not be thought of as mere hypocrisy nor its loving quality a sham. Far from it, a Cordelia-like tenderness can be quite genuine, but the preconditions for loving are incompatible with growth since they are both intensely possessive and subtly denigrating of their objects. Termination of analysis is quietly pursued as a fiat for a non-analytic and interminable relation to the analyst and to psycho-analysis. Needless to say, therefore, the configura-tion described in this paper is of special interest and concern for the analyst with patients who have a professional or social link with psycho-analysis.

In my experience, where the seduction of the analyst to idealize the achievement of pseudo-maturity, in its newly modified and 'analysed' edition, is firmly resisted, interruption of the analysis may be forced by the patient for ostensibly 'realistic' reasons. This may be done through engineering a geographical shift, a change in marital status, by promoting opposition from parent or marital partner, by contracting financial obligations which render payment for the analysis infeasible, etc., while still clinging to the idealized positive transference. If the analytic penetration is to succeed, a prolonged period of violently negative transference and manifest uncooperativeness must be expected and may prove intractable. This takes the form of injured innocence, self-pity, and the constant complaint that the analyst's implication that anal masturbation exists and continues in fact is either doctrinaire, a projection, or a manifestation of outside interference (e.g., from a supervisor).

Thanks to the constant clarification brought by dreams it is usually possible for the analyst to persevere. Gradually, by urging improved cooperation about consciously withheld associations and closer attention to body habits, the analyst can bring the hidden anal masturbation to light. With this the feeding-breast transference breaks through the restrictions imposed upon it by the idealization-of-the-faeces. Full-blown, painful and analytically fruitful experiences of separation anxiety become possible for the first time.

It is at this point in the analytic process that the relation to obsessional characterology becomes evident. The oscillation of the two states, pseudo-maturity and obsessional states, can be seen to take place, as the Oedipus complex in its genital and pregenital aspects takes the forefront of the transference. It can be understood that, for all the oedipal implications of earlier material which had required interpretation, a full experience of oedipal conflict only becomes possible when the differentiation of adult and infantile parts of the self has been thus arduously established.

Further Clinical Material

The clinical material which follows is intended to demonstrate the way in which strengthening of the alliance to good objects internally and to the analyst in the transference make possible a new stand against old anal habits. The patient in question came to analysis because of lack of direction in his work but analysis soon revealed also the pseudo-mature structure outlined in the paper. It also brought to light a little noticed continuation of anal habits and preoccupations which could be traced back in the anamnesis to nocturnal games with an older brother, probably never overtly sexual. But the unconscious splitting-off and projecting of a bad part of the self into the brother had played a large part in the self-idealization which underlay the patient's 'goodness' as a child. In fact the brother was by no means a bad child nor a bad sibling.

Approaching a Christmas holiday, the patient's recurrent fissure *in ano* became active again as the material swung toward patterns of anal intrusion into internal objects already well known by this fourth year of the analysis.

On a Tuesday, he reported having felt ill and cold since the unsatisfactory session of the day before. He dreamed that he was in a house with a man his younger brother's age and yet it was also the patient himself as a younger man.

This fellow seemed friendly and pleasant at first and was telling the patient that the bodies of police inspectors, often in a state of advanced decomposition, were being found all over Britain. Only when he indicated that there was one such in the next room under a sheet did the patient become alarmed. When the young man invited him to see it and the patient demurred, a tense situation arose. The patient backed toward the door and finally dashed out as the young man lunged for his throat. To his surprise there were policemen outside who reassured him that roadblocks were already established, and the young murderer would be dealt with.

In the second dream of the same night he found himself walking on the pavement, naked but for a tiny bath-towel, acutely embarrassed that his penis was visible. Thinking to get home more quickly and cut short the distress, he headed for a station, but was intercepted by a tramp who invited him to his nearby lodgings. He gladly accepted, but once in the tramp's bed he could not get to sleep, for the tramp stood upright by the bed all night and frightened him.

Note the contrast in these two dreams. In the first he is able to resist involvement in anal sadistic oedipal attacks on police-inspector daddies and finds himself comforted by the external relation to the analyst and analytic road-block process. But in the second dream oedipal humiliation in the bath-analysis drives him back to the anal preoccupation with a bad tramp-brother's faecal-penis in his rectum (the constipation which is a regular prelude to activity of his anal fissure).

On the Friday he complained of his constipation and noted that he had begun to diet in an obsessional way. An amusing incident had occurred the previous evening in which a 'fat' fly was buzzing about the house, finally landing on a vase. As he announced his intention to 'show the old gentleman to the door', picking up the vase with the sluggish fly on it, his young son wittily took the patient's arm and led *him* toward the door. He dreamed that he was waiting for a haircut in a queue, but it took so long, despite the fact that both man and wife were barbering on two chairs, that he despaired. Then he found himself lying comfortably in a little flat-bottomed boat going through a little tunnel (like one he'd been on as a child on a visit to Father Christmas at a big department store). When the boat was meant to make a right angled turn to the left, it became stuck, so the patient put his right hand into the water, making a scooping motion (as he had done the night before when the kitchen sink drain was blocked, to clear it). But he realized with a shock that his fingers were in the mouth of a tramp, lying in the water beneath the boat, who was about to bite him (anxiety about the constipation leading to the tearing open of his fissure, in contrast to the gentle 'showing-the-fat-old-gentleman-(fly)-to-the-door').

In this dream confirmation of the intolerance of separation (the couch-boat turning to the left; in fact when the patient leaves the couch it is *he* who makes a right-angled turn to the right) and turning to the tramp-faeces brother inside the mother's Father-Christmas-tunnel, is impressive. Note how the wish to rid himself gently of his oedipal rival (as his son's joke makes clear) leads him again to the alliance with the tramp brother, the constipated faecal penis and the tearing-open-the-fissure type of anal masturbatory defaecation. The infantile wish to make daddy old and expel him anally is still overpoweringly active, even though the patient's struggle against an abandonment to anal sadism has well commenced.

Three weeks later, on a Monday, he reported himself in a peculiar mood, full of intense and mixed feelings toward the analysis, aware that a recent insight helped him to curb a frequent type of provocative behaviour toward his wife but very worried and resentful about the coming holiday break. He dreamed that he was at a pond near my consulting room, waiting to go to his session. A man was fishing, though there are no fish in that pond, and had one of his two hooks stuck in the bottom. The patient had to free it, but was afraid the man would cruelly keep the line tight and cause the patient to be hooked. In fact this is exactly what happened. Determined to be free, he tore the hook out of his finger with pliers, tearing a piece of the flesh with it. To have it dressed he needed to go to a town outside London to see the American Ambassador. He was being fêted in a horse-drawn carriage before returning to the States; but, nonetheless, left the carriage and dressed the patient's finger and took him to his home. There the patient, feeling very happy, watched the Ambassador and his family have their lunch, separated from him by a perforated partition.

Here, before a holiday, the struggle to accept the oedipal distress (wound on his finger, linked to circumcision), and to free himself from the addiction to the anal masturbation (the man with his hook caught in the bottom on the pond, linked to the tramp-brother faecal penis) has proceeded with remarkable rapidity and clarity of insight. It is interesting that subsequently on two occasions he developed a paronychia of an index finger at week-ends.

SUMMARY

For the purpose of illustrating a current trend of our research into the intimate connexion between projective identification and anal masturbation, I have chosen to describe the transference manifestations of a type of character disorder seen with relative frequency among the many intelligent, gifted and outwardly successful people who seek analysis, namely of 'pseudo-maturity'. The concept of projective identification, first described by Melanie Klein, has opened the way to a new fruitful investigation of hitherto unexplored aspects of anality. By demonstrating how projective identification with internal objects is induced by anal masturbation, a richer conception of the derivation and significance of the narcissistic evaluation of faeces is unfolded, thus linking the anal phase more surely to symptom and character pathology.

Notes

1 Read at the 24th International Psycho-Analytical Congress, Amsterdam, July 1965.
2 Originally published in the *International Journal of Psychoanalysis*, vol. 47, pp. 335–342.

References

Abraham, K. (1920). The Narcissistic Evaluation of Excretory Processes in Dreams and Neurosis. In *Selected Papers* (1927). Hogarth.

Abraham, K. (1921). Contributions to the Theory of the Anal Character. In *Selected Papers* (1927). Hogarth.

Deutsch, H. (1942). Some Forms of Emotional Disturbance and Their Relationship to Schizophrenia. *Psychoanalytic Quarterly*, *11*, 301–321.

Freud, S. (1905). Three Essays on the Theory of Sexuality. In *SE* (Vol. 7). Hogarth Press, 1953–1974.

Freud, S. (1908). Character and Anal Erotism. In *SE* (Vol. 9). Hogarth Press, 1953–1974.

Freud, S. (1917). On Transformations of Instinct as Exemplified in Anal Erotism. In *SE* (Vol. 17). Hogarth Press, 1953–1974.

Freud, S. (1918). From the History of an Infantile Neurosis. In *SE* (Vol 17). Hogarth Press, 1953–1974.

Heimann, P. (1962). Notes on the Anal Stage. *International Journal of Psychoanalysis*, *43*, 406–414.

Jones, E. (1913). Hate and Anal Erotism in The Obsessional Neurosis. In *Papers on Psycho-Analysis* (1918 Edition, 2nd edn). Baillière.

Jones, E. (1918). Anal-Erotic Character Traits. In *Papers on Psycho-Analysis* (2nd edn). Baillière.

Klein, M. (1957). *Envy and Gratitude*. Tavistock.

Klein, M. (1957 [1946]). Notes on Some Schizoid Mechanisms. In Riviere, J. (Ed.), *Developments in Psycho-Analysis*. Hogarth.

Meltzer, D. (1963). A Contribution to the Metapsychology of Cyclothymic States. *International Journal of Psychoanalysis*, *44*, 83–96.

Rey, H. (1994). *Universals of Psychoanalysis in the Treatment of Psychotic and Borderline States*. Magagna, J. (Ed.), Free Association Books.

Spitz, R. (1949). Autoerotism. *Psychoanalytic Study of the Child*, *3*, 85–120.

Winnicott, D.W. (1965). *The Maturational Processes and the Facilitating Environment*. Hogarth.

Chapter 6

The Suffocating Super-Ego

Psychotic Break and
Claustrophobia[1]

A.A. Mason

SUMMARY

Mason examines the 'suffocating' super-ego and its role in claustrophobia and psychotic breakdown. He likens the omniscient suffocating super-ego to an attack of acute claustrophobia of the mind. He argues that claustrophobia arises as a defensive action against psychosis. To avoid an acute psychosis in analysis, Mason cautions against making premature interpretations and re-projecting parts of these unwanted projections back to the patient before the patient is ready to receive them. Deutsch (Chapter 1) argues similarly.

In distinction from the normal super-ego, this ego-destructive super-ego (Bion, 1959) contains the infant's catastrophic projections and is felt to be as dangerous and persecuting as the impulses it is intended to control. Suicide and psychosis might arise as a result of this persecutory and envious super-ego.

Citing Rosenfeld (1952, 1965), Meltzer (1973) and Bion (1959), Mason refers to the omnipotent, omniscient, and omnipresent super-ego. He invokes Bion's 'nameless dread' in the desired retribution of poisonous, cruel, ruthless, and remorseless emotions toward the object. Control of the object is pursued by the eyes in penetrating, relentless scrutiny and invasive, judgmental 'watching'. Esther Bick draws the same conclusion in her case material (Chapter 4).

Like Henri Rey (Chapter 7) and John Steiner (Chapter 8), Mason emphasizes the spatial component of no safe place for escape or shelter in the claustro-agoraphobic patient. Like Lewin (Chapter 2), Mason cites Poe's 'The Pit and the Pendulum' as a particular evocation of claustrophobic hopelessness and persecution accompanied by a crushing terror of no escape. Like Bick on different types of claustra (Chapter 4), Mason describes the terror of claustro-agoraphobic anxieties due to the projection of the primitive super-ego into an external claustrum. He emphasizes the varied geographical locations of the persecuting super-ego as occupying a somatic state in any part of the body, as in persecuting skin or the bowel.

Addiction in adults can follow the same developmental path as psychosomatic illness in infancy, as a result of claustrophobic, paranoid mother-infant pathological relating (in phantasy and in reality). We did not include the Case Histories 1–3 or "A Note on Psychosomatics" due to space limitations.

DOI: 10.4324/9781003200284-6

TEXT

Introduction

This paper is an expression of gratitude to Dr. Wilfred R. Bion, who supervised the first psychotic patient I treated by psychoanalysis eighteen years ago. His support and understanding helped me to complete a successful analysis of that case. This encouraged me to continue the psychoanalytic treatment of psychosis in ten further cases, eight of which continued analysis unto completion.

One of the findings of this experience is presented here with the hope that another generation of analysts might be encouraged to pursue the treatment and investigation of these disorders.

The Suffocating Super-Ego: Psychotic Break and Claustrophobia

This paper has arisen from my experience with two different clinical problems: First, the acute psychotic breakdown arising spontaneously or in the course of psychoanalysis. Second, the treatment of claustrophobia.

I found at times that these two apparently separate clinical problems unexpectedly turned out to be different facets of a similar problem. Patients who develop psychotic breaks suffered anxieties, symptoms, and defenses which had a marked similarity to those experienced by patients who had been treated for acute claustrophobic anxiety. Similarly, these claustrophobic patients frequently developed symptoms and anxieties of a psychotic nature. This, quite often, was especially noticeable when the claustrophobic anxiety diminished.

Detailed examination of the core dynamics of both these groups of patients has led me to believe that at times claustrophobia arises as the result of a defensive action against a psychotic breakdown, and a central issue is the type of super-ego structure present. It is to this particular super-ego quality that the substance of this paper is addressed.

The Super-Ego

The upright stance and the development of speech, along with the presence of the super-ego is one of the attributes of man that has raised him above the animal kingdom. This structure is responsible for his conscience, his morals, his ethics, his religion, and his esthetics. It is the source of all his spiritual aspirations and endeavors. However, the super-ego has also a side that becomes man's enemy, for as well as protecting and inspiring him, it punishes, tortures, reviles, and can destroy him. In fact, a great deal of our life is spent either in following the dictates of the super-ego or attempting with varied success to escape them. Freud (1923), who first described the super-ego, called it the heir to the Oedipus complex, its derivative, and its substitute. A child between the age of three and five, faced with the impossibility of his Oedipal wishes, because of his love for his parents and his fear of punishment, permanently incorporates and installs these parents inside his mind. This internal image of them has now become an internal object, which continues to live and act inside the child's mind, controlling, threatening, or punishing it whenever its Oedipal wishes attempt to make themselves known. Melanie Klein (1933) continued Freud's investigation into the nature of the super-ego and her work expanded our understanding of it through her exploration of the early processes of introjection and projection. She developed Freud's idea that Oedipal super-ego was an installation of the image of the parents in the ego, and showed that this internal structure grew continuously by additional introjections from the outside world. Mrs. Klein also showed that the introjections which form the super-ego were not simply reflections of external reality, but contained also the child's projections into them. Thus the objects which formed the super-ego were a composite of external reality plus infantile projections.

Once this point was accepted, we came to realize that the infant's own contributions to the nature of its super-ego are as important and at times more important than those of the external world. Freud himself was puzzled by the exaggerated and distorted image the child had of his parents, and never satisfactorily explained it. Freud's view of the harshness of the super-ego was based on three ideas: 1) It was due to the individual's harsh aggressiveness turned against himself. 2) It was a continuation of the severity of the external authority. 3) It was based on the primal-horde father of prehistoric times. Mrs. Klein drew our attention to the early feelings of the child which are violent, uncontrolled and often too terrifying to contain. These feelings are then treated in the way that the child treats all frightening and intolerable internal states, and that is to project them into the outside world and into its objects.

The success of this manoeuvre is, however, limited; for at times the external terrors can themselves become so overwhelming that the child now reintrojects them in an attempt to control them. This process of projection and introjection and reprojection and reintrojection may be repeated over and over again in an attempt to deal with internal and external persecution. The formation of the super-ego is one result of this defensive process. The normal super-ego becomes the controlling agent of the dangerous id impulses but the abnormal, or excessively destructive super-ego, i.e., that super-ego containing the infant's destructive projections, becomes itself felt as dangerous and as persecuting as the impulses it is supposed to control. Many disastrous consequences may follow in the presence of such a persecuting super-ego and the internal dynamics are reminiscent of the nation-wide students' rebellion of the late '60s and early '70s. The students, under the belief that the establishment was oppressive and would not give them their due, or even listen to them, marched against their own colleges, smashing, looting, and destroying. The colleges and police attempted to suppress them, often using great force and violence. This produced even greater explosions of rage and frustration from the students and the situation grew increasingly violent and uncontrolled. One could say that psychosis had taken over.

When the super-ego is felt to be harsh and persecutory, it, too, may lead to a revolution of the ego and id impulses that are being crushed by it. A breakdown or breakup of the personality may follow where parts of the ego and the id are fragmented and projected with great violence. Sometimes the super-ego itself becomes the victim of the rebellion and is thrown out of office and projected into the outside world. When these fragmentations and projections occur clinically, they manifest themselves as psychotic breaks of a schizophrenic or manic type. This process has been described fully by Rosenfeld (1952). In attempting to avoid and in the treatment of this catastrophe, it is imperative to understand the nature of the formation of the persecutory super-ego, so that one can modify it, and the effects it produces.

The literature contains many papers that describe the severe, harsh, murderous and persecuting nature of the super-ego. In particular, those of Mrs. Klein (1927): She put forward that the super-ego existed much earlier than Freud described, and dated it at the beginning of the Oedipus complex and not as the heir to it. She also dated the Oedipus complex itself at the weaning stage of infancy.

This early super-ego is formed by the introjection of terrifying figures produced in fantasy by the child's sadistic impulses toward its object. In "The Psychoanalysis of Children," Klein (1932) suggested that introjection begins at birth and the incorporated object immediately assumes the function of a super-ego.

In 1952, she added to her concept of the super-ego as a persecutor by describing in great detail the formation of the envious super-ego. In 1957, she had a change of view and stated that the super-ego develops with the two instincts, life and death, in a state of fusion and that the terrifying internal figures which result from intense destructiveness do not form part of the super-ego proper. They exist in a separate area, in the deep unconscious where they remain unintegrated and unmodified by normal processes of growth. These terrifying figures may in situations of stress infiltrate and overwhelm the ego. Mrs. Klein suggested that in the splitting-off of these frightening figures, de-fusion of the life and death instincts is in the ascendency and these extremely bad figures are not accepted by the ego. She also related these persecuting objects to dead and injured objects. Meltzer (1968) elaborates on this aspect of the super-ego introjects later.

Whether these early and terrifying figures are called primitive super-ego or are seen as totally apart from the super-ego, I fully agree with her idea that the presence of anything which strengthens them or allows them to in infiltrate the rest of the mind is an important factor in psychotic breakdown.

My own observations suggest that there is something in the quality of these early internal figures that needs further elaboration. As Mrs. Klein wrote in her paper on the early development of the conscience,

> The child's fear of his objects will always be proportionate to the degree of his own sadistic impulses. It is not, however, simply a question of converting a given amount of sadism into a corresponding amount of anxiety. The relation is one of content as well.

The particular aspect of this content which I have observed cannot be described simply and I will attempt to explain it by describing several of its facets. One such facet has been studied extensively by Rosenfeld (1965), Meltzer (1973) and Bion (1959) and may be described as omnipotent, omniscient, and omnipresent. The common factor is the word "omni" meaning "all," thus: all-powerful, all-knowing, all-present. This super-ego quality creates a sensation in the mind of being watched by eyes from which nothing can escape. These eyes are cruel, penetrating, inhuman and untiring. They record without mercy, pity, or compassion. They follow relentlessly and judge remorselessly. No escape is possible for there is no place to shelter. Their memory is infinite and their threat is nameless. The punishment when it comes will be swift, poisonous and ruthless. An important effect of the omnipotent super-ego is the production of feelings of hopelessness which can result in either suicide or psychosis.

The hopelessness is engendered particularly by the feeling that the merciless, implacable quality of the internal watcher cannot be defied. Struggle against it is useless and resistance is futile. Added to this feeling of being constantly watched and threatened there is also the sense of being acutely listened to, smelled, and even having one's thoughts read, which gives some idea of the terror and hopelessness produced. These sensations create in the subject of their implacable scrutiny a feeling of being totally surrounded by irresistible forces which close in on them from all sides like the Iron [Maiden] of medieval tortures or the contracting room of Poe's "The Pit and the Pendulum." This particular form of persecution may not only cause a feeling of hopelessness in the subject, because of the belief engendered that no escape is possible, but the crushing and suffocating quality also produces panic and explosion, in a desperate attempt to escape, even at the cost of disintegration. The internal effect of the omniscient suffocating super-ego could be likened to an attack of acute claustrophobia of the mind.

Meltzer described the quality of paranoid anxiety that I am concerned with as terror, and believes it to be due to dead objects, particularly dead internal babies. Meltzer believes that the anxiety produced by these dead internal babies has an inescapable quality. He also described one outcome of the terror, which is a submission to the tyranny of a bad part of the self which promises to protect one against the terror. I fully agree with Meltzer about the importance of the inescapable quality of persecution of the super-ego but in addition to the consequences described by him believe that it is this very quality of the terror that produces anxiety of an explosive kind, which is extremely important in the formation of psychotic breaks. Moreover, I believe that when panic and psychotic breaks occur, it is because the persecution has become worse than inescapable, it has become suffocating and devouring. It therefore produces a violent reaction equivalent to that which occurs when respiratory obstruction or the fear of being eaten is experienced by any living organism, particularly as these two anxieties often occur simultaneously.

What are the roots of this implacable monster? The answer surely must originate in the equally implacable phantasies of the helpless infant, who is in reality so weak and so totally unable to defend himself, that his only weapon is his mind, aided by his organs of perception. So, all-powerful, originally, means the infant's all-powerful phantasies directed toward its primary object, the mother, or her breast. The child's controlling phantasies are strengthened by the use of a particular omnipotent mechanism described by Mrs. Klein (1957) as projective identification, where parts of the self are projected into the object, for many purposes, particularly to possess and control the object.

Mrs. Klein described the use of oral, urethral, and anal phantasies for this purpose. I believe that in addition to this, the organs of perception are of particular significance in this mechanism. The senses such as hearing, seeing, and smelling can all be used in phantasy to put parts of the self into the object as distinct from receiving perceptual stimuli from the object. This now imparts to the phantasy a controlling quality of great power. This process was first described by Bion (1958) in "On Hallucination." The capacities to see the object at a distance, to watch its every movement, to follow it around with one's eyes, all strongly support the feelings of omnipotent control. One even has the capacity to shut it out, i.e. annihilate it, by closing one's eyes, and bringing it back by opening one's eyes and letting in the light, just like God. The mere blink of an eye creates or destroys in phantasy one's objects. "Let there be Light!"

Hearing, too, can support phantasies of omniscience powerfully, not only because it supports sight, but also because it can function in the dark when sight is not possible. Hearing the parents speak, thus always knowing where they are and what they are about. Hearing them in bed and in intercourse all support phantasies of taking part in these activities, invading them and controlling them. The open door of the child's bedroom permits phantasies of control by hearing, as the night light gives it phantasies of control by seeing. Smell, too, allows the belief of taking part in the mother's activities, and the capacity to smell the breast is probably present from the beginning of life. Later on, smelling other bodily secretions can give the infant the belief that it is in contact with the intimate parts of the parents' bodies.

I see you, I hear you, I smell you, really means I touch you with my eyes, ears, and nose, and if I touch you I can hold, possess, and control you. In addition to these manoeuvres, there is also the phantasy of getting inside the mother with the senses; and seeing, hearing, and smelling take on the additional significance of knowing. To "know you," to "know about you," to "know all about you," contains always the phantasy of power and control over "the object." "Knowing," in this kind of phantasy means more than being acquainted with, it means in possession of. Knowing in Biblical terms means carnal knowledge, i.e., intercourse, and the knowing I am describing is very close to this in sense. It implies a penetration of the most intimate parts of the object, and therefore in phantasy controlling and possessing the object. "I see you," "I know you," "I know all about you," "I possess you": if one says and listens to these words, the sense and feel of their underlying phantasies become plain to us. "Knowledge" becomes power indeed in the child's mind.

I have already mentioned oral, anal, and urethral phantasies of affecting and controlling the object and would like to expand again on the quality of these phantasies. The child's cries are meant to affect the mother, but often in phantasy are meant to do much more than that. The piercing, the penetrating cry associated with the phantasy of control, and often the phantasy of projecting parts of the self into the object is believed and hoped by the helpless infant to possess and tie his mother to him. "I hear and I obey" is the phantasy counterpart that we and the object are meant to respond with. Sometimes the object does respond in just that fashion, following its own unconscious hope that when in the past it called imperiously or desperately, it had to be answered. The stark realistic fact that no one may be there, or even that if they are, they are not compelled to answer, is too frightening for the immature ego to tolerate. There is no single word that describes these invasive voyeuristic, listening and smelling phantasies, but when I describe invasive voyeuristic control, I am implying that senses other than sight may be used, sometimes separately and sometimes together, in the service of possessive invasion of the object.

The function of stools and urine in controlling the object is well documented, but I would like to add a note about the phantasies that stools and urine are frequently felt to be the object or part-objects themselves. The thumb-sucking child, as Freud (1941) observed, has the hallucinatory wish fulfillment that he possesses the breast or, as he wrote in his last words "is the breast." Mrs. Klein, expanded Freud's idea, and would have said that the child utilizing the phantasy of projective identification has projected its empty mouth into the breast and taken possession of the nipple, which it now holds in phantasy in its thumb, and can administer to itself. This nipple possessed and surrounded by the child's mouth, trapped and controlled, in fact virtually devoured, will later, when introjected into the ego, become a super-ego component which will be felt to surround, trap, devour and suffocate the child's personality in phantasy, producing the internal claustrophobia and acute psychotic breaks previously described.

Each of the three claustrophobic patients I have treated demonstrated marked oral fixation. One sucked his thumb from early babyhood to the age of 19, when he replaced it with cigarettes. Another could not be detached from her bottle and comforter until the age of 6 or 7. Even today, at the age of 57, she cannot venture out without candy, pills or breath mints in her bag, which still comfort and protect her.

The constipated stool may be similarly phantasied as the trapped nipple, felt to be now devoured and held and controlled, sometimes sadistically, in the rectum. Later, when it is introjected and installed as a super-ego component, it returns its former treatment to the infant's mind "with a vengeance." A patient had the following dream while suffering from an acute bout of constipation. "The King and Queen of England were held prisoner in the Tower of London in a dark airless dungeon. I would watch them through a small hole and think 'How have the mighty fallen.' One day, I went to see them and found they had been released-the dungeon was now filled with sun and air and was empty. I knew with a feeling of dread and panic that it could only be a question of time before they returned to become the head of the State and would throw me into an even deeper dungeon from which I could never escape."

These physical activities of sucking, crying, urinating, and defecating, and many others are thus added to the sensory activities, looking, hearing, etc., described previously, and together with phantasies of omnipotent and omniscient control help the child modify its feelings of extreme helplessness in relationship to its object.

The phantasies all give it the belief that the movements and life, inner and outer, of the mother are monitored, watched, and controlled, i.e. virtually devoured. In fact, the object is felt to be so trapped that not even a breath can be taken without the child's wishing it to be so. It is particularly this feeling, of not being able to breathe, which adds a quality of panic and desperation to the persecution that is conducive to fragmentation and breakdown.

It is certain that the infant's early perception of its primary object is not only a breast and nipple, but something that has the sound and movements of a living organism, particularly the sound and movements of respiration, as the child is held so closely to the mother's chest a great deal of the time.

When phantasies of controlling this primary object occur, they may become linked initially to phantasies of controlling the respiratory movements as well. I believe that this quality of breathing control, plus the quality of devouring the object, when re-introjected and installed as a super-ego component, adds to the already suffocating anxiety produced by the omniscient and voyeuristic components of the super-ego previously described. These four components – omniscience, voyeurism, devouring phantasies and breathing control – together make for a suffocating quality which is the cause of intense internal anxiety and which produces the tendency to rupture and explode.

Now, there are eyes, ears, and a nose inside of oneself, watching acutely over one's every movement and hearing one's every sound as well as a mouth holding one trapped and ready to swallow one. Added to all this is an omniscient quality which penetrates into one's deepest layers, knowing all about one's every activity, and holding one trapped and suffocated by this knowledge. This internal figure reminiscent of Orwell's Big Brother in the novel *1984* watches, and threatens continuously and also suffocates as it prevents any movement.

It is this feeling of having no freedom, no exit, no escape, that simulates the feeling of being unable to breathe, the mental equivalent of which, like all sensations of respiratory obstruction produces a violent panic, internal rupture and explosion-the psychotic break. Therefore, it is the roots of this feeling, i.e. the infant's intense, suffocating, omniscient, controlling and devouring phantasies and activities toward the object, and toward the analyst in the transference, which have to be minutely analyzed for relief to be obtained. I believe Bion hinted at this in *Elements of Psychoanalysis* (1963). When the intrapsychic strain caused by the suffocating super-ego becomes intolerable, psychotic break due to fragmentation of the ego is probably the most extreme consequence that may follow.

Other consequences or what may be called defenses against this strain that I have observed are as follows:

1   The use of drugs of all sorts, to blanket and dull the persecution of the super-ego. In fact, many drug addicts originally became addicted because they used their drugs as a self-administered treatment of the anxiety produced by the persecution of their super-ego. One could say that the addict who takes drugs to deal with the intolerable inner-tension caused by a suffocating super-ego is effecting the kind of therapy for himself that he often would get if he went for psychiatric treatment. Sometimes the drugs administered by psychiatrists are less harmful than those self-administered, but at times they are identical. Alcohol, heroin, the hypnotics and barbiturates are used frequently by patients for this purpose. It follows that taking these patients off drugs without adequate analysis of the persecutory anxiety will not only be futile, but will at times actually precipitate psychosis. It is even worse for some of these patients to be taken off drugs and confined to a hospital or prison, as this compounds the feeling of claustrophobia by adding a real external suffocation to the internal one. In such situations not only is psychosis a danger, but suicide may be attempted in a desperate endeavor to escape their terrifying feelings of suffocation.

2   The all-seeing, all-knowing super-ego may be projected into outer space where it becomes the "God of Wrath" of the Old Testament. Presumably He can then be handled more easily by worship, placation, or merely because there is now more distance between Him and the self. I believe that the religious conversions experienced by many adolescents in particular are their attempts at solution of the suffocating tension suffered by them through their primitive super-ego. This religious conversion is sometimes an alternative to the drug solution, sometimes it accompanies the use of drugs, and sometimes it supersedes it.

    One of my patients became extremely religious and orthodox during adolescence: in his words, "more orthodox than the priests." During his infancy, he was extremely controlling to his maternal object, both through direct demands and a chronic psychosomatic illness. Among his first words as a child were "get it" accompanied by an imperiously pointing finger. During adolescence he spent years "getting it" for God and being frightened and depressed if he felt that he had failed to please Him in any of His wishes. His psychosomatic illness was asthma, which trapped his mother at times in phantasy and fact, and then in turn, following projection and reintrojection, trapped him inside his own chest.

3   Fragmentation and projection of the super-ego into the patient's objects can also occur. This results in persecution of the "ideas of reference" type. The belief that one's mind is being read, that one is being controlled at a distance, that one is being hypnotized, all can be the result of the projection of the omniscient voyeuristic super-ego into one's objects and experiencing the "all knowing control" now being in them and being exerted toward oneself.

Two patients of mine occasionally projected their suffocating super-ego into their spouses. When this occurred, they both experienced intense feelings of suffocation when in contact with their wives. One could not bear any physical contact with his wife at all. Love-making was impossible and panic producing, and even sleeping in the same room was difficult to tolerate. His wife's breasts were experienced as "buffeting his face" and he had to break away dyspneic and panic stricken. He had been a thumb sucker until the age of 19-trapping and "suffocating" the nipple in his mouth constantly. His bouts of promiscuity with "unknown" women and even occasional homosexual episodes were totally in the service of escape from the feelings of suffocation that his wife's body produced. On analysis it could be demonstrated that she had become the receptacle into which his suffocating infantile mouth had been projected. This patient's anxieties seemed to date from as far back as feeding during infancy for according to his mother he would choke when he fed from her breast until her doctor advised the use of a nipple shield through which her nipple protruded during feeding. When I recall how this patient would thrust his way into my office, sometimes bumping into me on the way: and how his voice bored into my head and his eyes penetrated me with a steely blue glance, I had little doubt that the nipple shield prevented him from asphyxiation because of his invasive thrusting into the breast. I often longed for the psychic equivalent of a nipple shield during sessions when he bore into my mind. From the patient's point of view the thrust was experienced the other way round, and he complained about my thrusting interpretations down his throat, and recalls how his mother "cornered" him in the morning with a bowl of cornflakes, and how suffocated he felt by her "pushing the food at him."

Another patient spent his weekends as a "cowboy roaming freely on the prairies," imagining he was free from any responsibilities, wife and children, all of whom made him feel asphyxiated. At times he became suffocated by the smog of the city and would drive furiously into the country to be able to breathe freely.

This patient had a long history of intensely possessive behavior toward his mother and many years of chronic constipation. When analyzed, his stools in phantasy were sometimes the breast and nipple of the maternal object, and sometimes the father's penis, swallowed or taken in per anum and trapped and held in his rectum. When he had periods of diarrhea, the trapped nipple and penis in phantasy were now expelled and experienced as either "smog" in the air or earthquakes on the ground threatening him. Both these phobias produced intense claustrophobic anxiety and attempts to run out of town and away from them.

On one occasion, I believe a psychotic break was narrowly averted by the analysis of his failure to pay his bill, which was unconsciously equated with trapping me in his "bank-rectum." He simultaneously developed great anxiety and persecution about the demands of his wife, children, and business, particularly in terms of financial demands, and felt annihilated and suffocated by them. He felt driven mad and talked about suicide as an escape from these impossible debts and demands.

It was finally the analysis of his withholding of money from me and the phantasies of what this was doing to me which enabled him to pay his bill, i.e., let go of me and a subsequent diminution of internal and external persecutory tension resulted.

A third patient who projected her super-ego into me during a session jumped out of my second-floor window in a panic, as she felt too acutely suffocated to get out of the house by the slower route of stairs and door. She had been an extremely controlling child, mainly using illness to attach her mother to her. She also had a history of being four weeks in an incubator after birth, having been born prematurely. She had many memories and dreams, all describing an intense and controlling attitude toward breast, chest, and respiratory movements of her maternal object in me. Frequent dreams of persecution contained large animals breathing heavily which pursued her. Although there was a sexual element in the heavy breathing, it was also a return of a persecutor which now attacked her with its breathing. Internally she frequently experienced her own feelings to be too heavy and too violent to bear; this produced feelings of suffocation and panic. (Compare Dora [Freud 1905] who also had asthma and was intensely controlling to her objects, maternal and paternal.)

4   Another common consequence of the suffocating super-ego is the production of the familiar symptom of claustrophobia.

Freud (1900) described a phobia as a projection and displacement onto an external object of inner conflicts which are causing a disturbance in the ego, so that the danger of developing anxiety now threatened not from the direction of an instinctual impulse but from the direction of a perception.

Melanie Klein (1946) related claustrophobic anxiety to the fear of being imprisoned inside the mother, following phantasies of invading and attacking the mother's body, using the mechanism of projective identification. Joan Riviere (1948) spoke of claustrophobia as due to a fear of retaliation following projective attacks on the object. Gehl (1964) linked claustrophobia to depression and en passant to paranoia and drug addiction, although he does not spell out the details. He does, however, confirm my own observations about the common occurrence of asthma and respiratory habits in conjunction with claustrophobia. My view that claustrophobia is both an internal state linked to persecutory super-ego phantasies of a suffocating nature and an external state brought about by the projection of this super-ego into an external claustrum encompasses and develops both Freud's and Klein's ideas. Klein seems to be describing a consequence following the projection of a split off part of the self into an object. She does not continue with the consequences of this primitive phantasy when the object is now introjected and forms part of the super-ego.

The claustrophobia I am describing, i.e., that due to the projection of the suffocating super-ego into an external claustrum, is a much more organized and detailed phantasy when analysed clinically. The claustrums commonly used are planes, elevators, crowds, cinemas, dentists, hairdryers, etc.

All these things in external reality which of themselves can shut in and hold one confined can have the persecuting element of suffocation added to them by the projection into them of the super-ego qualities previously described. One claustrophobic patient once actually heard his father's voice in his head admonishing him, and after shaking his head "saw" his father's stern face in the outline of a mountain. This produced extreme feelings of being trapped and threatened by the mountainside and caused him to drive away in panic. Just as having one's God outside, it is no doubt more tolerable to have one's claustrophobia outside. There, one can attempt to flee from it, while if it is inside, it is inescapable.

5   In 1960, while conducting a research project for the Asthma Research Council of Great Britain on the psychotherapeutic treatment of asthma, I noted (1962) that three patients treated by me converted to claustrophobic anxieties after the remission of their asthmatic symptoms. The symptomatology changed from their chests to their minds, but the anxiety of being suffocated remained the same.

Since then, I have analysed four asthmatic patients and have noted that there were strong oral fixations in three of them. All had great difficulty in separation from their primary object, the breast. Later in their lives, the breast became equated with their inhalers which they also could not be separated from and which they carried constantly with them, trapped in their mouths or pockets. This "breast-inhaler" in its turn, after introjection, trapped them mentally as a super-ego component. It was then projected into their bronchi where it changed into asthmatic attacks which now suffocated them physically. Consequently, I believe that some asthmatics, particularly those characterized by broncho-spasm as distinct from swelling of the bronchial mucosa, fall somewhere in between the claustrophobias and the psychoses.

A conclusion of these findings would therefore be that the occurrence of certain types of asthma (consequence S), the production of claustrophobia (consequence 4), like the worship of God (consequence 3), the production of paranoia (consequence 2), or the use of drugs (consequence 1), can all be defenses against psychosis. It also follows that extreme caution must be exercised in the analytic treatment of claustrophobia, as the return to the patient of those parts of the self-projected out in defense may produce acute psychosis. The underlying anxiety must be elucidated, interpreted, and traced back to its origins, for the projected aspects of the personality to be accepted back safely. This is also true of all patients in whom psychotic breakdown is a danger.

I would also like to differentiate between the anxiety produced by the particular suffocating super-ego quality I have described, and the discomfort experienced whenever any form of concrete thinking is present in the patient.

Concrete thinking frequently arises as a result of the use of massive projective identification by the patient when concretization is present, fusion with the object is also present in phantasy, and the mind does not think about the object, it thinks the object instead. Instead of the infant thinking about the breast, its thoughts are the breast. This omnipotent phantasy that the thoughts are the object produces a subjective feeling in the mind of a space occupying lesion. In contrast, thinking which is an abstract phenomenon does not produce the feeling of something literally present. The mind which literally thinks the breast becomes squeezed out of existence by the breast it has omnipotently produced. Subjectively this often produces a very uncomfortable feeling which is described variously as a pain in the head, a headache, a stuffed feeling, or other statements indicating the feeling of having two objects competing for one space. Sometimes a feeling of drowsiness is present, confusion is common, and associated symptoms of depersonalisation, unreality and deja-vu phenomena are often present. In the most severe cases fragmentation and projection of this state of mind can occur. The patient typically cannot symbolise and literal thinking in which thoughts are felt to be identical with physical actions is present. Segal (1957) described this in her paper "A Note on Symbol Formation."

In contrast, the feeling accompanying the suffocating super-ego is invariably associated with a trapped sensation. The distress is similar to that produced by respiratory obstruction, accompanied by a wish to break out or break loose, panic frequently supervening. Concrete ideation is usually absent. The patient typically is anxious, distressed and agitated, cannot stay in one place and feels that he is jumping out of his skin.

SUMMARY

A particular quality of super-ego is described which can produce an anxiety of a suffocating nature. This anxiety is produced by certain kinds of super-ego components acting together or separately. Four of these components have been described.

(1) Omniscience (omnipotence and omnipresence)
(2) Voyeurism (visual, auditory and olfactory elements)
(3) Breathing Control (control of respiratory and other movements, control of dangerous gases)
(4) Devouring (oral-trapped nipple, anal-trapped stool)

All these components are installed into the super-ego by the infant using the mechanism of projective identification which because of its omnipotent invasiveness imparts an invasive quality to the super-ego.

The consequences of the suffocating anxiety produced by the super-ego described are as follows.

(1) Psychotic Break: Fragmentation and projection out of ego and id. Sometimes fragmentation of super-ego.

(2) Drug Use: Self or psychiatrically administered. Relieves tension between super-ego and ego and id.

(3) Projection Outward of Super-ego:

   (a) Into the sky – Religious conversions.

   (b) Into one's objects – Paranoid relationship of suffocating nature – frequently leading to divorce or child runaway.

   (c) Into inanimate objects – Elevators, crowds, planes, etc. Typical claustrophobia.

   (d) Into body organs (somatisation) – Bronchi – Asthma; Bowel – Colitis; Bladder – Frequency; Blood vessels –Hypertension, Raynaud's disease.

Symptomatic treatment of (2) and (3) a, b, c, d may produce psychosis. When a psychotic break threatens, the patient's monitoring suffocating phantasies toward the analyst in the transference have to be traced in great detail and dissected carefully back to the underlying primitive anxieties producing these defences.

The transference present when this dynamic is in evidence is frequently of a nature I would like to call voyeuristic. Here the patient comes to the analysis in order to watch, observe and "know all about" the analyst rather than his own state of mind. Material is produced to see how the analyst deals with it and to learn about the analyst's mind, and about psychoanalysis, in place of getting analysed. The patient's emphasis is on the examination of the analyst's secret shortcomings and not on his own. Excitement and feelings of power are produced by these observations, just as with the voyeur, and the patient's "cure" is to become a psychoanalyst, leaving the analyst as the patient.

Note

1 Editor's Note: In this contribution Dr Mason has significantly pinpointed an internal object which is common to psychotics, asthmatics, and other psychosomatic patients. He believes the object causes claustrophobic anxiety and is characterized by omnipotence, omniscience, and omnipresence by virtue of the projective identification of omnipotence generally and of the qualities of the sense organs particularly into an object, which is thus internalized in this awesome manner. In particular, he believes that the fragmentation that leads to psychosis is the result of an anxiety which *is* a psychic equivalent to the panic experienced when respiratory function is threatened. In a separate contribution, I wrote about the *magus*, which I believe to be an internal object characterized by eerie, sphinx-like sorcerer qualities and composed of the projective identification of the epistemophilic instinct from the patient. I believe Dr Mason is describing the same or similar object from another vantage point and is thereby casting a rich clinical light on a powerful internal enemy.

References

Bion, W.R. (1958). On Hallucination. *International Journal of Psychoanalysis*, *39*, 341–349.

Bion, W.R. (1959). Attacks on Linking. *International Journal of Psychoanalysis*, *40*, 308–315.

Bion, W.R. (1963). *Elements of Psycho-Analysis*. Heinemann.

Freud, S. (1893). Draft B from Extracts from the Fliess Papers: The Aetiology of Neurosis. In *SE* (Vol. 1). London: Hogarth, 1966, pp. 179–183.

Freud, S. (1900). Interpretation of Dreams. In *SE* (Vol. 4).

Freud, S. (1905). A Case of Hysteria. In *SE* (Vol. 7).

Freud, S. (1918). An Infantile Neurosis. In *SE* (Vol. 17). London: Hogarth Press, 1955. pp. 1–122.

Freud, S. (1923). The Ego and the Id. In *SE* (Vol. 19).

Freud, S. (1925). *Inhibitions, Symptoms, and Anxiety*. In *SE* (Vol. 20). London: Hogarth, 1959.

Freud, S. (1941 [1938]). Findings, Ideas, Problems. In *SE* (Vol. 23). London: Hogarth, 1964, pp. 299–300.

Gehl, R.H. (1964). Depression and Claustrophobia. *International Journal of Psychoanalysis*, *45*(2), 312–323.

Klein, M. (1927). Psychological Principles of Infant Analysis. *International Journal of Psychoanalysis*, *8*, 25–37.

Klein, M. (1932). *Psychoanalysis of Children*. Hogarth Press.

Klein, M. (1933). Early Development of Conscience in the Child. In *Contributions to Psychoanalysis*. Hogarth Press.

Klein, M. (1946). Notes on Some Schizoid Mechanisms. In *Developments in Psycho-Analysis*. Hogarth Press.

Klein, M. (1952). On the Theory of Anxiety and Guilt. In *Developments in Psycho-Analysis*. London; Hogarth Press, pp. 271–291.

Klein, M. (1955). On Identification. In *New Directions in Psycho-Analysis*. London: Tavistock, pp. 309–345.

Klein, M. (1957). *Envy and Gratitude*. Basic Books.

Mason, A.A. (1962). Asthma. *British Medical Journal*, *11*, 371–376.

Meltzer, D. (1968). Terror, Persecution, Dread. *International Journal of Psychoanalysis*, *49*, 396–400.

Meltzer, D. (1973). *Sexual States of Mind*. Scotland: Clunie Press.

Poe, E.A. (1842). *The Pit and the Pendulum*. Penguin Classics (2009).

Riviere, J. (1948). Paranoid Attitudes in Everyday Use and in Analysis. *Lecture to the British Psycho-Analytic Institute*, 1948.

Rosenfeld, H.A. (1952). *Notes on the Analysis of the Superego Conflict in an Acute Schizophrenic*. Tavistock.

Rosenfeld, H.A. (1965). *Psychotic States*. Hogarth Press.

Segal, H. (1957). Notes on Symbol Formation. *International Journal of Psychoanalysis*, *38*, 391–397.

Chapter 7

The Schizoid Mode of Being and the Space-Time Continuum (Before Metaphor)

Henri Rey

SUMMARY

Henri Rey was born on the island of Mauritius and worked for many years at the Maudsley Hospital in London. He coined the term 'claustro-agoraphobic dilemma', which gave the title to this book. In his work with severely disturbed schizoid and borderline patients (Rey 1994), he discovered that many of them could tolerate neither intimacy nor separateness. They lacked a stable sense of identity and therefore tried to enter an external object like a shell or an exoskeleton. Inside the object, they often felt encaged and imprisoned. Outside, they felt abandoned or feared falling apart. More than any other psychoanalyst after Sigmund Freud, Henri Rey was interested in the spatial dimension of the human mind. He linked Melanie Klein's ideas about unconscious phantasy and the two 'positions' with Jean Piaget's research on the development of early 'sensori-motor schemas'. In his view, biological and psychological births do not coincide since the infant, like the newborn kangaroo in his pouch, lives for a while inside the mother's mental space before he can develop his own mental space and differentiate it from the external world and the internal space of others. Rey received impulses from the work of Joan Rivière, Herbert Rosenfeld, and Hanna Segal (see Steiner 1994). He was also interested in mathematics and psycholinguistics and observed that schizoid patients often used words in a concrete way like 'things' or 'acts'. This connects to another important focus of Rey's work: the difficulty of schizoid patients to symbolize and repair the damaged figures in their internal world (Rey 1984, 1988). Rey's discoveries continue to be further explored and expanded by analysts like John Steiner (see Chapter 8 in this book) and other psychoanalytic writers.

TEXT

The Schizoid Mode of Being

The period that followed the Second World War revealed a remarkable change in the kind of patients seen by, or referred to, the psychotherapist and the

DOI: 10.4324/9781003200284-7

psychoanalyst. The bulk of patients seemed to consist of a certain kind of personality disorder which defied classification into the great divisions of neurosis and psychosis. We now know them as having a borderline, narcissistic, or schizoid personality organization. This simplification is the result of a long process of attempts at classification of all kinds.

An attempt has been made in this essay to extract aspects of human behaviour and mental processes that seem to constitute the core of what we now know as schizoid or borderline personality organization. It can be found not only in those people with such a personality as will be described, but also in people who may break down into schizophrenia, depression or mania, or as the underlying core of personality in people with hysterical or obsessional personality. By studying the schizoid traits in these various states, I hope to be able to define the schizoid personality and the schizoid mode of being in its more or less pure form, and to distinguish it from the other states of which it may form part. It seems that those people represent a group who have achieved a kind of stability of personality organization in which they live a most limited and abnormal emotional life which is neither neurotic nor psychotic, but a sort of frontier state.

Schizoid and/or borderline patients when seen by the psychiatrist are usually in their early twenties. They complain of an inability to make contact with others, and find it impossible to maintain any warm and steady relationship. If they actually manage to enter into a relationship it rapidly becomes intensely dependent and results in disorders of identity. They rapidly and transiently form an identification with their objects, and experience a loss of their sense of identity with the self. They seldom establish a firm sexual identity, and vacillate in their experience of maleness and femaleness. They are not homosexuals but have fears that they may be, and their choice of love objects, or attempts at choice of love objects, are just as vacillating. They are demanding, controlling, manipulating, threatening and devaluing towards others. They accuse society and others for their ills and are easily persecuted. This may be associated with grandiose ideas about themselves. In fact, their feelings are dominated by phantasies of relative smallness and bigness. When threatened by feeling small and unprotected and in danger they may defend themselves by uncontrollable rages and various forms of impulsive behaviour.

Other aspects of their abnormal affectivity are reflected in the sense of futility they complain of and which is characteristic of them. This is reflected as well in the special kind of depression from which they suffer, a form of depersonalized depression, that is, boredom, uselessness, lack of interest, with a marked deadening of the pain aspect of true depression. Together with this deadness there is a search for stimulants and production of sensory experience by means of alcohol, drugs, hashish, cutting themselves, perversions, promiscuity. They often complain of various abnormal sensations, body-image disturbance of various kinds, as well as depersonalization and derealization experiences. Their body ego is no more structured and stable than their personality, ego or self. Their underlying state of perplexity and confusion is frequently apparent.

Their work performance varies a great deal. Often when they come to treatment they have given up their studies or their work or they are doing some form of manual or low-level occupation, although they may have achieved university standards. However, their working capacity may be preserved if they work in a structured situation.

There is one difference in my personal experience in the way the two sexes present themselves, with many more men responding to the description I have given than women. In the case of women, hysterical manifestations – that is, hysterical mechanisms of defence – mark the underlying personality structures, and they show more often than men histrionic behaviour, acting out, hysterical fits, and overtly the claustro-agoraphobic syndrome. The claustro-agoraphobic syndrome, however, is basic to both sexes; only certain manifestations of it are different. As Guntrip (1968) has so clearly described, the schizoid person is a prisoner: he craves love but is prevented from loving because he is afraid of the destructive force of his love so far as his object is concerned; he dares not love for fear that he will destroy. He finds himself enclosed in a dilemma, enclosed in a limited space, and with limited objects and limited relationships.

It is the mechanism at work in this 'limitation state' that I intend to describe. Kindness and support in the transference situation are not enough to treat these patients. A thorough knowledge of their mental processes, phantasies, and underlying structures subtending their behaviour is essential, in combination with affective understanding.

I will begin with internal part-objects and their language – projective identification – because we must begin somewhere in this Tower of Babel which makes up the schizoid structure. I mean this expression literally because these part-objects whose structure we need to understand speak to each other and speak to us in a confusion of languages which demand special interpretation.

In normal interpersonal relationships one or another aspect of the whole ego corresponds with one or another aspect of the ego of the other person. It is a relationship at the level of the integrated ego. Moreover, in normal conduct, apart from certain aspects of love and hate, when we tend to be concrete, the ego makes use of conventional signs which are conscious and of symbols which may be conscious or unconscious, both, however, existing at a representational level.

Schizoid communication by contrast often takes place at a level of 'merchandise', a sort of barter agreement in which the subject feels himself to be given 'things', made to accept 'things', and where 'things' are done to him. Thus, after weeks or even months of refusing to speak of her intimate feelings a patient said, 'You don't understand. If I speak to you I hit you. I poison you with the rotting and mouldy things which I am full of.' She had previously simulated a suicide attempt in order to get her stomach washed out, to clean out some of these contents. Another patient said, 'When you speak to me and ask me questions you bite me and tear out a piece of my flesh. I won't speak anymore, I won't listen.' It is a well-accepted fact for psycholinguists that at first the utterances of the mother are considered to be experienced by the child as perceptual parts of mother like any other parts.

Moreover, more or less normal people think in terms of persons, not objects placed somewhere in a container. In contrast, this is just how schizoid thought functions: thoughts are material objects contained somewhere and expelled into something or other; even the containing object is itself contained somewhere. It is thus that the schizophrenic is the patient who most concretely shows the true problem of claustrophobia and agoraphobia. In the consulting-room he sits near the door or the window even if this cannot be opened sufficiently for him to escape. He feels himself to be engulfed, immured in one object or another, and feels that he does the same thing with the objects which are inside him.

A schizophrenic patient illustrated this by explaining why he was frightened to lie on the couch. He was afraid of becoming engulfed in it, and, being so tall that his feet overlapped the couch, he feared that his father would see his legs poking out and cut them off. He could not distinguish between the couch and his mother in his unconscious phantasy, and felt himself caught inside his mother with only his feet showing. This is concrete thinking, where the idea is equivalent to the object and where these idea-objects are always contained or containing.

We must now consider the characteristics of these objects and their fate when they are displaced. This will lead us to examine the notion of partial objects, and of splitting and denial. It is remarkable that these ideas, which took on an increasing importance in Freud's thought, remained unused, or almost so, by the adherents of classical psychoanalysis. To quote Laplanche and Pontalis:

> It is of some interest to note that it was in the field of psychosis – the very area where Bleuler too, from a different theoretical standpoint speaks of Spaltung – that Freud felt the need to develop a certain conception of the splitting of the ego. It seemed to us worth outlining this conception here even though few psychoanalysts have adopted it; it has the merit of emphasizing a typical phenomenon despite the fact that it does not provide an entirely satisfactory explanation of it.
>
> (1973, p. 429)

Similar comments could be applied to the concept of partial objects and of denial since these concepts are interdependent. I think it is necessary to make an important distinction between a pathological part-object and a normal part object, which is only partial in the sense that it forms one of the parts of an object which is capable of being assembled into a whole. Thus the maternal breast is a part-object only by comparison with the whole mother formed by the integration of her various parts, and functions in an infant phantasy like an object endowed with capacity for action, love and hate.

Splitting plays a part in normal development also, for example, splitting of good and bad aspects of the object as well as of the subject, and also the splitting of one object from others. But the schizophrenic behaves differently. Under the sway of persecutory anxiety and the fear of catastrophic dissolution of the ego – primitive and elemental anxieties which arise from the beginning of life – he proceeds to use splitting repetitively and intensively to get rid of bad parts of himself, which leads to a fragmentation of the object and of the fragmented parts of the ego, as well as fragmented parts of internal objects. The impulses and anxieties belonging to these fragments are projected into his objects, which acquire by projective identification these split-off aspects of the self, now projected and denied. These objects become persecutors and are introjected, but cannot be assimilated. They are in turn projected into an external object – or even into an internal object in an intrapsychic relation – and the vicious circle continues. These objects, some of which Bion has called 'bizarre objects', are important as elements in the thinking not only of the schizophrenic but also of the schizoid patient. These processes do not only apply to bad aspects of the object or of the self: from fear of destruction, the good parts of the object or the ego are also split off and projected in the same manner into objects which are expected to look after them while they contain them, preserving and protecting them.

In the course of psychotherapy, the schizoid, having projected his good parts into the therapist in order to preserve them, as if depositing them in a bank, becomes frantic if he cannot find his therapist, which would mean also the loss of elements of the self and of his objects. Moreover, since the reparative activity of the schizoid is based on concrete reparation, as if he were rebuilding a house with its bricks, the loss of the 'bricks' contained in the therapist makes reconstruction impossible. This, in my opinion, is one of the fundamental reasons for the schizoid's refusal to form an ordinary transference relationship with the therapist. Unless one can interpret this mistrust, which is fundamentally justified and which the therapist needs to understand, it is extremely difficult ever to obtain the confidence of the schizoid patient. Concurrently with these internal splits, the therapist too is split into good and bad objects, and the transference relationship changes constantly and remains unstable and fragmented for a long time, changing not only from day to day, but from minute to minute during the session.

Thus, a young schizophrenic whom I treated in hospital perceived me either as an object whom she could not do without – from whom she could not separate, and to whom she wanted perpetually to adhere – or, within an instant, as an object which she attacked so vigorously that I had to defend myself from her by force. One day she illustrated the change from a neurotic transference to a psychotic transference in a remarkable way: she spoke to me about her life at home in a reasonable manner and in contact with reality, and then, all of a sudden, with astonishing rapidity, she went to the door and with piercing eyes and voice trembling with emotion she said, 'Get down here in front of me. Obey. You know how for years you have mistreated my mother and me, the cruelties and torture that you have done, when you came to my room at three o'clock in the morning.'

External reality had disappeared and only psychic reality remained. The image of the father and of me had become one. I had become her father with his partly real characteristics and those partly attributed to him by the patient by that same process of projective identification. At the end of five minutes, which seemed as long as five centuries, when I wondered what was going to happen, she became calm and resumed a more or less normal conversation. But she remained mistrust-ful, close to the door, as if she might await the return of the 'feared ones' which she called 'they', and which would come to take her away to a hellish fate. She could not be friends with me because 'they' became angry and punished her. It was best to be on good terms with 'they'. She asked if she could kill me to con-vince 'they' that she did not love me. On the other hand, the idea of losing me was intolerable: after she let down the tyres of my car so that I would be killed in an accident, she hid herself to watch me, and ran after me to warn me that if I went in the car I was in great danger, without telling me why.

The fear of separation from the object and the desire to penetrate into it and fuse with it into a primal unity can be so intense that it surpasses human under-standing. Thus, a paranoid and persecuted patient complained ceaselessly with years of virulent reproaches full of rage and despair because I did not love her, after having seduced her by my interpretations and having led her to believe that she was loved. She found proof of my wish to torture her in the fact that I did not let her penetrate into me physically and fuse with me. On this subject she lost all contact with reality and insisted that such a fusion was possible. One proof of my refusal, which made the analysis almost impossible, consisted in reproaching me as often as she could that I was not in agreement with what she was saying. This produced two people, not one person, and I became a monster which, at least at that moment, she hated.

It is clear from what I have just said that the question of his or her identity is a major problem for the schizoid. The enormous difficulty of acquiring a stable ego is the result of faulty introjective identification, made very difficult by per-secutory feelings and a fear of the object created by the projection of destructive, envious, and insatiable impulses, which can become incredibly violent. They are neither heterosexual nor homosexual, not even bisexual. This arises from the fact that their identifications depend both on an internal object which is not assimi-lated, and on a containing external object in which they live; hence this identity depends on the state of the object and varies with it, its identity and its actions. They have an external shell or carapace, but no vertebral column. They live as parasites in the shell which they seem to have borrowed or stolen, and this creates a feeling of insecurity.

Thus, an extremely schizoid young man, who during his treatment went through a breakdown diagnosed by all the psychiatrists except me as totally schizophrenic, would dress himself at night in clothes typical of a London businessman. He would enter his parents' bedroom at three o'clock in the morning, wake them and say to his father, 'Am I now the person you wanted me to be?' Previously he had dressed himself in his mother's clothes for a number of years. Under the pressure of the psychotherapeutic group where he received treatment, which attempted to confront him with his lack of initiative and his failure to leave home and go to work, he decided to become a man.

One day, some workmen happened to be working on road-works in front of his house; he urinated into a bottle, which he put at the front door as a gesture of contempt. He looked at himself in a mirror, brushed his hair in the style of Wellington, and in a military manner marched around the courtyard. He then took some of his neighbour's washing, which was drying on the hedge between their houses, and threw it into her garden. He invited the workers to tell him who gave them permission to be there, and then returned to his house. Since it was the first of May, a special day for workers, he sang a patriotic anti-Communist song. Then he convinced himself that he was in danger because the workers were Communists and would attack him. Moreover, the BBC would begin to talk about him, and the Irish rebels would come to get him. He had become important, but persecuted, and his homosexual passivity and his feminine identification entered into the conflict as a passive defence. Finally, to separate himself, to undo the identification with his parents, he became irritable, oppositional and aggressive. They could no longer look after him, and he was admitted to the hospital as an in-patient.

During individual sessions with me he sat on the floor to look up at me from a lower position as a sign of respect, like a baby. Then he said that if he lay down, or sat down, he would, like a baby, fail to orientate himself in relation to the things around him. Later, he became preoccupied with multiple aspects of his personality: he no longer knew which parts of his parents he was made of, and each piece had a nationality: his father English, his mother German/Polish, now living in England. Each 'piece' had a special and separate characteristic. His father is a professor, but in addition was a military man through family tradition, but at the same time a pacifist; he is upper- and lower-class, conservative and socialist, and so on. He began to believe that his mother was Jewish. He gave a nationality to a large variety of 'pieces' including one 'piece' of him that was Prussian, and very rigid, one 'piece' that was English, and one 'piece' Polish. Then he wanted to become a Jew, and soon after he changed his mind. First he admired them, then he criticized them. Finally, he explained to me why he wanted to become Jewish: it was because the Jews were fragmented, dispersed, persecuted and dispossessed, living in a Tower of Babel of languages and of different nationalities, and yet found their unity and their identity by the fact that they were Jewish, a fact that could transcend and unite all these fragments into an integrated whole.

What a marvellous unconscious description of the integrative functions of the object! He had to have this schizoid regression, this dissociation of parts which had been assembled in a faulty way in order to separate out the elements and to reconstruct the edifice. This example illustrates clearly the problem which integration of the ego poses for the schizophrenic or schizoid person.

Schizophrenic Breakdown

I have had the occasion to treat a young schizophrenic who had an attitude resembling catatonia, and very interesting rituals in which a gesture of her limbs or face was always annulled by an opposing gesture controlling and undoing the preceding one. I eventually understood that these gestures were either sexual or aggressive and needed to be controlled. After the death of her father she adopted typically catatonic postures and said she could not move because she would come into collision with her father, who was enclosed inside her.

Later, with other patients, I came to understand that the opposite of immobility could be seen in paroxysmal movements such as those of an epileptic fit, which by contrast results in the projection of internal contents outside, where they can be attacked and destroyed. Then I came to understand the extreme mental rigidity of the schizoid who has to control all his objects, both internal and external. The anxiety of his sexual persecutory and destructive impulses is so great that no autonomy can be allowed to his objects. The fear of fragmentation is catastrophic. Thus, a schizoid man could alter nothing of his life or his attitudes, and said he could never live anywhere else than at his home because if he moved he would have to take with him his room with all his furniture and things as they were, without changing anything.

Transformation, Representation and Symbolization

The second fact to consider with the schizoid is the mental apparatus necessary for the transformation of sensory or sensori-motor experience into representations, into images, into symbols and signs, and into memories – such transformations being essential both for the maintenance of ordinary human relationships, and for the construction of a normal mental apparatus for thinking.

We have seen that the elements of thought in the schizoid have a concrete character which Freud himself described as one of the essential qualities of the system Unconscious, namely, the representation of things instead of the representation of words. This defect in the function of transformation seems to be a basic defect in the schizoid. But at the same time we know that the schizoid is in many cases capable of great intelligence-even though he treats people as things, thus removing the affectivity which for him is dangerous and persecuting. The coexistence of a schizoid type of personal relationship and of a highly developed intelligence can only be explained by a split in the ego which results in a partial ego, which is intellectual and highly developed such as Piaget or Hartmann would describe, and another part of the ego in which the development has been arrested at the schizoid stage, and where the depressive position has not been worked through.

During psychotherapy with the schizoid, progress in treatment depends on the possibility of undoing this schizoid structure and of allowing normal symbolization of bizarre objects and of sensory experiences to occur; that is to say, to make other modes of communication possible. It is sometimes possible to achieve this without a catastrophic reaction – without the coherent parts of the ego disintegrating. In other cases this is impossible and the patient needs to go through a frankly schizophrenic episode. For some this is a good thing because it is the only way of returning to the point of bifurcation between normal and abnormal development where the growth of a paralysed affectivity, previously enslaved and rigidly controlled, may be resumed. If this happens I believe no one can predict whether the patient will become a chronic schizophrenic or will progress towards new horizons.

The same situation applies to the schizophrenic in a clinically obvious schizophrenic state: does he have the potential to resume his development or not? This chiefly depends on the capacity of his mental apparatus for symbolic transformation and on the stage he has reached in relation to the depressive position. Indeed, there is a group of patients for whom the schizoid state is a regression and constitutes a defence against the suffering and pain of the depressive state; these patients have a better outlook than those who are true schizophrenics, those who have never reached the depressive state. A schizoaffective state, whereby the patient oscillates between a state of schizophrenia and depression, is also well known, and these cases again have a more favourable outcome with psychotherapy. We also know of cases which without treatment change from schizophrenia to depression or vice versa in the course of time.

Among those who have studied the function of transformation and representation in the mental apparatus, the work of Bion (1965) stands out as especially significant. I would like to give an example of defective transformation. Bion says, 'In psychoanalytic theories statements by patients or by analysts are representations of an emotional experience. If we can understand the process of representation this will help us to understand the representation and that which is represented.'

A patient told me the following dream:

> I am dining with friends and get up from the table. I am thirsty and I start to drink. I realize that the bottle in my mouth has a neck shaped like a feeding bottle; there is no teat, but I think I can feel the flange which normally holds the teat in place. While I think of this I begin to see the bottle more clearly, I hold it in front of my face and see that it has the shape of a feeding bottle. In the bottle I see water. The level of the water falls and bubbles of air mount through the liquid, and because of this I am aware that some of the water has become part of me; but I cannot feel this thing that becomes part of me. I am anxious because I can neither understand nor feel the water passing from a state separate from me to become an intimate part of me. While I am thinking thus, the bottle becomes bigger. I see at that moment that on the inside of the bottle facing me, words are engraved on the surface in raised letters which give instructions on how to wean an infant.

In this dream the subject failed to transform the experience of the movement of water from the exterior to the interior of his body into a good experience in the form of a representation and a memory. He did not participate in the experience; he did not understand what happened; he tells us that he lacks the experience of the change. This can only be the experience in the mouth where the presence of water produces a sensation, a sensation which is needed to make the work of transformation possible. One part of the experience is lacking; it is as if he had been fed through a tube. But he tells us what was lacking – it was the teat and it was the experience of weaning, and of suckling from a mother. He took the bottle himself and gave himself a drink. The teat no doubt represents a maternal breast and a mother whose presence and whose bodily contact is absolutely necessary for the awareness and recording of the experience. It seems that in the absence of the good object, part of the work of assimilation did not take place.

Reparation

In addition to structural mechanisms of the schizoid phase and its mechanisms of defence I would like to consider a fundamental aspect of schizoid mentality. This is the law of the talion and the absence of the capacity for reparation which governs the whole behaviour of the schizoid. By the law of the talion I mean: an eye for an eye and a tooth for a tooth; let the punishment fit the crime; if I have stolen, my hand will be cut off, if I have transgressed I will be punished, you have stolen and I will cut off your hands. It is this law of vengeance which is responsible through its incredible power in the schizoid not only for the stunted mental structure, but also for its lack of humanity. There is no forgiveness, no compassion, no reparation. There is only the terrible vengeance and anger of Jehovah as preached by the prophets of the Old Testament.

Reparation in the schizoid state also obeys the law of the inverse talion. Like everything I have already described, it has to be concrete. I call this repair to distinguish it from reparation; we could also perhaps call it reconstruction, which has some things in common with the restitution with which Freud was concerned. Reparation, on the other hand, is a notion unknown to Freud and plays a fundamental role in the work of Melanie Klein. Even Freud's ideas on restitution remained sketchy and far from complete, as were his ideas on splitting and denial. Almost all analysts have rejected the fundamentally new theme which appears in his work after 1920 in which the life instinct as a constructive force was contrasted with the death instinct as an instinct of disintegration. People have quarrelled about words and have forgotten that analysis is rooted in observation. The study of the schizoid personality structure has led us back to the observations of a master on splitting, projection and denial, which Freud's ultraconservative disciples had well buried. In reconstruction or repair, infantile omnipotence is retained and an attempt is made to reconstruct the damaged one. Reparation, by contrast, is not and cannot be an omnipotent act.

The Manic Defence

We will now consider the role of the manic state. On the one hand its role is a defence against the anxiety of disintegration and of schizoid persecution, and on the other hand a defence against the pain of the depressive state. One can observe this from the point of view of psychiatry in the clinical syndrome of hypomania, but also as a potential psychodynamic state during psychotherapy. We must not forget that the manic state can represent an exaggeration of a normal phase of maturation and of reparation. I believe that in all depressive states the object with which the subject has a relationship is, contains, or symbolically represents the maternal breast, which as a partial object represents the mother who is destroyed, emptied, or poisoned, and thus is in a depressed state. The subject feels this is his fault, becomes identified with this depressed object, and consequently depressed himself.

In manic states or in the manic defence we are no longer concerned with the maternal breast but with the penis. The object of the manic state is the penis which is needed by the subject for the task of reparation: through it he can regain the destroyed object either as a direct substitute by identification or by recreating the contents of the mother, for example, by making her pregnant by filling her empty breasts and so on. The more the maternal object is destroyed by the subject's attacks, the more must the penis become omnipotent, and the subject by identification becomes omnipotent also. In this manner the destroyed state of the object is denied. There is no reparation proper, and after the manic phase the subject returns to his depression or his schizoaffective state at the level of maturation which he had previously reached.

A very schizoid patient dreamed that on his nose he was balancing a long pole which reached right to the sky with a baby balanced on the end. As he awakened he said to himself, 'This fucking penis is good for nothing, it's so big that it's useless.' On the couch, the patient (of whom I have already spoken) had identified his whole body with a phallus, and felt himself to enlarge physically and be invaded by delusions of grandeur. In the manic state we have a pseudo-penis which repairs nothing; it serves to deny the reality of destroyed objects, and presents itself as the universal substitute, which leads to the formation of a false self. Meanwhile, the aggressive impulses continue to destroy the object.

Manic reactions can actually represent a pathological deviation of a normal phase of development. I believe that when the separated fragments of the ego reunite, whether in a mosaic or in a fusion, it is done with the help of the phantasied action of the phallus. This is achieved on the one hand by an identification with the penis, adopting its characteristics and functions; and, on the other hand, because, although a partial object, it usually functions, as we have explained, as a representation of the whole object – the father – and enters into the relationship with the maternal breast, the partial object representing the mother. We have here the prototypes of the sexual identity of the two sexes and the prototype of the relationship between them. The role of the penis as a creator integrating and repairing through reproduction becomes clear in this model.

However, in the manic state there is a partial identification with the immeasurably grandiose aspect of the erect penis. The manifestations of this aspect are omnipotent, contemptuous, and persecutory as well. It is always present in a latent form in the schizoid, and, when seen clinically as delusions of grandeur in paranoid states or as a feature of the depression of the manic-depressive, illustrates the role of the phallus in the grandiosity seen in these conditions.

The patient referred to earlier, who felt himself to vary in size both physically and mentally, explained that he felt he had a permanent personality for the first time when he experienced the presence inside him of a hard column extending from his anus to his mouth, which could resist all attacks. Later, in his grandiose state, he identified with Jesus Christ, grew a beard and became a carpenter, designed religious motifs and wanted to preach in church.

The Depressive Position

It will not be possible to go into the mechanism by which a depressive state develops, even though this forms an essential phase in treatment. This is work about which much has been written, and I want to concentrate on schizoid states. Suffice that we remember that in this process destructive impulses lose their intensity and loving impulses play a fundamental role. The good and the bad parts of the ego and also of the object unite gradually into a whole, and the law of the talion loses its virulence. Primitive compassion begins to take over from the total egocentricity characteristic of the beginnings of life. The object achieves a life of its own, and the subject becomes an object related to like any other object.

From Schizoid States to Schizophrenia

These phases of development belong to the preverbal period. Instead of the basic development, we have here to understand a triphasic evolution: first an archaic preverbal phase and an archaic verbal phase where the distinction can be thought of as an example of ontogeny repeating phylogeny; then, after the age of six, seven, eight, a phase in which external reality dominates. I take the view that non-verbal schemata give a structure to verbal thought, which in turn influences the pre-existing non-verbal schemata. This reciprocal relationship sheds light on the disorders of verbal thought which are seen when a schizoid individual becomes schizophrenic. The task of defining what happens when this change from a schizoid to a schizophrenic state occurs is not easy; the more I understand the language and structure of the schizoid the more I find the distinction difficult.

From the point of view of classical psychiatry it is quite simple: are there delusions or hallucinations? If there are, it is schizophrenia, if not, it is not. But when one works not only longitudinally but simultaneously in depth as the psychoanalyst does, the situation is quite different. We can see this if we compare material from schizoid patients with the delusional ideas of someone floridly schizophrenic.

Let us take an extreme case, a patient who had four schizophrenic breakdowns, each presenting a different clinical picture. In his hebephrenic catatonic state, which began with an intense interest in the universe and the stars, he felt himself to be communicating with an extraterrestrial universe. As proof he took out of his briefcase some little oval- and circular-shaped pieces of ivory-coloured paper, and assured me that their extraterrestrial origin was obvious. Much later he admitted that although at first he had firmly believed this, he later came to realize that he himself had simply collected these pieces of paper from somewhere.

We see here the interplay of a number of schizoid mechanisms. First of all, the wish to be omnipotent, to participate in the universe, which he held very strongly. To achieve this wish without becoming mad he had to avoid destroying external reality and instead tried to transform it. With the external physical proof he could thus reinforce the internal psychic reality of his wish. For this he had transformed the pieces of paper through the phantasy of projective identification and obtained in this way a formal proof of his experience. He had thus decided not to abandon external reality completely, but grossly to transform it by a process of splitting, by omnipotent wishing, and by projective creation.

Some schizoid patients are past masters in the art of choosing objects which are precisely appropriate for their projections; that is, which have characteristics so similar to their projections that it becomes very difficult to make a distinction between the object and the projected phantasy.

It seems to me, then, that the schizophrenic goes further and does not concern himself with the existence of external reality, but declares and delusionally believes whatever he wishes, having made a regression to a very primitive, infantile stage where the distinction between psychic reality and external reality is almost non-existent and hardly concerns him. There is only one reality – the reality of the internal phantasy world. In the schizoid world we find various gradations of abnormality in the type of morbid processes I have just described.

The Space-Time Continuum and Displacement in the Borderline

An attempt will be made now to examine the clinical observations previously described, in terms of the organization of space and time as in any other branch of knowledge. Piagetian observations, ideas and constructs have been extensively used both explicitly and implicitly but by no means exclusively. The main source for this work is clinical observation during treatment and psychoanalytical psychotherapy supervisions, and interpretations of data. I have made use of Piaget only for the reason that psychoanalysis has never studied the structure of external reality – of space, displacement and time – as have he and his pupils.

During the treatment of patients, especially of claustrophobic and agoraphobic patients, it appeared more and more evident to me that a fundamental organization of objects in space (including the patient himself) was underlying the mode of behaviour observed. All sorts of physical and mental situations which claustrophobic and agoraphobic patients experience are very likely to refer to a primary situation which all the other secondary situations are substitutes for and symbolic of.

Claustrophobic persons are afraid to be in an enclosed situation; they develop extreme anxiety or panic and want to get out. The 'situation' may be a room, a traffic-jam, a marriage. When they are not contained, they become agoraphobic and develop anxiety or panic. Thus they may be housebound, or may only travel so far alone from the place of safety and no further, or have to be accompanied. The manifestations of those conditions are well known. However, it was when I made the observation that this condition is really a basic one in schizoid states and schizophrenia that I realized it had a very important meaning. By a basic condition I mean that whenever schizoid and schizophrenic patients are seen in the context of dynamic treatment they reveal claustro-agoraphobic basic fears not in the least evident when their behaviour is assessed from a purely phenomenological psychiatric approach. The mental and emotional disturbances of the schizoid state are disturbances in the early, primitive and basic organization of the human being, ontogenetically speaking. It is the importance that Piaget gives to the early structuralization of space that led me to attempt the explanation of the way of life of the schizoid in terms of the early organization of space, movement and time.

Spatial Development of the Infant and His World

The foetus is at first contained within the uterus, which is itself contained inside the mother. It is relatively deprived of freedom of movement and displacement, although a certain degree of movement is possible. It moves with the mother in the mother's external space. After birth, one could say that the mother through her care, feeding, warmth and support recreates partially this uterine state for the baby. Although restricted still, the baby's personal space allows him more freedom than in the womb. It could be called the marsupial space. The baby now moves in the mother's space, but only in that portion of her space which is the baby's personal space. As he or she grows up, the personal space increases until it has coincided with the maternal space. If the mother is normal, for instance, not claustro-agoraphobic, that space will coincide with general space, where the subject will be an object among objects. Simultaneously with this process a space internal to the subject is formed where psychic internal objects live in intrapsychic relationships. They are experienced very concretely at first, for example, as sensations, or elaborated later as representations of a very complex nature.

It would seem that everybody has an external personal space of some kind which persists, somewhat like the notion of territory in ethology, and in which our object relations are somewhat different from those in the universal space. However, as Piaget has pointed out and described so clearly, space is not a Newtonian absolute space, neither is time absolute time; they are both constructs. The infant and the child have to construct their objects and their space, space being the relative positioning of objects as in the Einsteinian model,

The idea, then, would be to look at some aspects and stages of those early constructions and how they appear either unevolved or distorted as structures underlying the schizoid mode of being. The pure Piagetian approach is unsatisfactory, for although emotions, affects, and drives are accepted as intrinsic parts of the cognitive structures, they are not referred to as such. I will therefore present my own psychoanalytical and Piagetian inspired elaborations.

Objects that are familiarly looked upon and treated as individual wholes by adults are certainly not experienced as such for the infant. The child has to 'construct' them, linking parts by action schemas as described by Piaget, that is, by interiorized actions of the subject on the object. Piaget says the child co-ordinates

> . . . the actions among themselves in the form of practical schemas, a sort of sensori-motor preconcept, characterized by the possibility of repeating the same action in the presence of the same objects or generalizing it in the presence of analogous others.
>
> (Battro 1973)

For Piaget more complex schemas are not just the association or synthesis of previously isolated elements. Thus, he writes of the sensori-motor scheme that

> . . . it is a definite and closed system of movements and perceptions. The schema presents, in effect, the double characteristics of being structures (thus structuring itself the field of perception or of understanding) and of constituting itself beforehand as totality without resulting from an association or from a synthesis between the previously isolated elements.
>
> (Battro 1973)

For Piaget the 'sensori-motor schemas are not simply what we sometimes call patterns, that is to say, they have further power to generalize and further power to assimilate' (Battro 1973).

As to schemas relative to persons, Piaget says that 'they are cognitive and affective simultaneously. The affective element is perhaps more important in the domain of persons and the cognitive element in the domain of things, but it is only a question of degree.' Thus, he says that an 'affective schema' means simply the affective aspect of schemas which are otherwise also intellectual.

For Piaget, action is at the very beginning the source of all manifestations of life. It precedes thought, it controls perception and sensation. It is by a process of combinations of actions of the subject on his object, followed by the internalization of these action schemas, that the precursors of thought are generated. Thus the infant puts his or her thumb in the mouth, then extends this action to other objects, then elaborates the action by using a rod or some such object to extend the reach of his or her arm to get to objects that will be taken to the mouth or elsewhere.

I do not know if a study has been made of such a way of thinking in Freud's writings apart from the structural theory itself. But it is interesting to note that in the Rat Man, for instance, Freud makes constant references to psychical structures. In fact, Part IIa is entitled 'Some General Characteristics of Obsessional

Structures' (Freud 1909). He says that 'obsessional structures can correspond to every sort of psychical act', and:

> In this disorder (obsessional neurosis) repression is affected not by means of amnesia but by a severance of causal connections brought about by a withdrawal of affect. These repressed connections appear to persist in some kind of shadow form (which I have elsewhere compared to an endopsychic perception) and they are thus transferred, by a process of projection, into the external world, where they bear witness to what has been effaced from consciousness
>
> (p. 221)

This is as good a definition of mental structure as any structuralist could wish.

For the object-relations psychoanalyst, therefore, there exists in the behaviour of adults primitive object relationships or schemas, normal or pathological, which govern aspects of behaviour. Some of these primitive internalized object relations may have remained unintegrated and function autonomously. Part-object psychology, or the psychology of part-object, part-subject, part-states, relates to the study of the aspect of the genetic development of object relationships.

Starting with the need of the infant expressed as desire for gratification, there is little doubt that the infant wishes to make part of his endogenous space, that is, the precursor of the self, the gratifying objects he needs for survival and growth. His early discovery of the appearance and disappearance of the object in his space (early ego or self) will prompt him to desire the good objects as part of himself or of his good space in the only way he is capable – the concrete. The frustration of not being able always to keep the object in his spaces (that is, internal space and personal space) will increase the desire for the object to be his possession. The growth of this desire and the need for securing such objects, if it reaches great intensity, will become greed. The frustration, anger and anxiety resulting from the non-possession of the desired gratifying objects will lead to the desire to deprive it of the other space containing the desired objects, for the other space containing the objects is now in a state of no-pain or pleasure, a state previously experienced by the infant. The wish is not only to possess the object, but to deprive the other space as he is himself deprived. This is envy.

Further, the infant left in his self-space while waiting for the gratifying object will have to substitute objects of his own self-space, for example, parts of his own body or toys. Thus in the place of the breast-mother he will have thumb, excrements or genitals as part of his space. They may prove helpful in waiting for the appearance of the external breast-mother, and thus temporarily relieve anxiety or frustration following non-gratification. Non gratification may lead to punishing the non-self-space by putting frustrating objects, say faeces, into it, thus substituting them for the good breast or transforming it into a bad object. However, those parts of the self-space put into the non-self-space are still considered to be somehow part of the self-space, and a particular kind of bond is formed between self-space and non-self-space by displacement in or out of them – that is, by introjection and projection. This bond gives to early object relationships a quality of possessiveness and identification between objects which are at the roots of introjective and projective identification processes.

This process is by no means abnormal when it is concerned with displacement of objects for need gratification and communication purposes. Its persistence and distortions are, however, responsible for a large number of typical features of the schizoid way of experiencing. It creates the feeling of living in the object because part of oneself is in the object; it creates the need for never leaving the object out of control; it creates a sense of impending doom through the possible loss of part of the self if the object is lost. And it results in persecutory feelings if the projected or displaced part of the self is believed to have envious, greedy, and destructive impulses, and accounts for innumerable other schizoid manifestations,

We shall now proceed with the systematic examination of schizoid manifestations in terms of our space-time model, and illustrate this with examples. First of all, I will try to show how one must extend the claustro-agoraphobic syndrome from a specific syndrome to a basic universal organization of the personality. A claustrophobic woman is seen for assessment for psychotherapy. She says she is afraid that something terrible will happen to her if she goes out. She insists she does not know what it is. I point out that there are only two possibilities, either it is something she will do to others, or something others will do to her. She says after a lot of hesitation, 'I'm afraid I'll do something mad.' After more hesitation, she says, 'I'll shout and people will think I'm mad.' I say, 'Shouting is something coming out of you. What else could come out of you?' She becomes extremely tense and nervous, and after a while asks to be allowed to leave. I say that, of course, she can leave if she so desires, but if she can have the courage to say what thought is making her so uncomfortable that she wants to leave, it might save her months of treatment and misery. She plucks up the courage and says, 'Urine and faeces.' I will leave out the rest of the interview. This is a routine happening in various forms.

What years of study of my own patients and patients treated by others has revealed I will put in schematic form. It will be noticed that the patient wanted to remove herself from the space where she was in contact with what she felt as a threatening object. She wanted to leave the room. However, we also know that phobics avoid certain situations, for instance, eating in public; they will not go to a restaurant, or to the cinema, or to shops. They restrict their outside space until they are housebound. It is important to understand what the ultimate space into which they retire corresponds to in the unconscious.

The outside world or outside space is in such an instance transformed by projective identification into the body or internal space of the subject him or herself, identified with the internal space of the mother. Thus entering and coming out of a room is coming out of that which the room stands for ultimately – the mother's body. A primitive imprinted state of birth experiences persists in the hierarchies of transformation and representation of that early experience. What is fixed in the mind is not necessarily the original experience of birth, but one or another experience of a primitive similar state belonging to the hierarchy of space constructions, such as the marsupial space described previously. When something comes out of the body such as a shout, urine, faeces, semen, saliva, or vomit, it fires the system coming-out of and produces the attached affect. The mechanism involved is the identification by projective identification of the subject with the contents of his own body, and of his body identified with that of the mother; he thus experiences himself coming out of the mother.

As I have said, the primitive emotional experience, the affect, has been dominant in the structurization of the self- and the non-self-spaces. Displacement, then, of any kind of objects, including the subject himself from self-space to non-self-space or vice versa is experienced in a primitive manner. Space in certain circumstances is experienced as it was once experienced in a part of the personality, split off from the rest, and this way of experiencing space persists. The panic associated with that state and the bodily anguish and sensations are but the persistence of the experience when the ego was mostly body ego. The coming into activity of that split-off archaic part of the adult self takes over and paralyses the more adult ego. Thus adult methods of coping with danger are no longer available.

I realized the fundamental structure underlying all this when I came across the same experiences as a basic state with schizophrenics, for example: their difficulty lying on the couch from fear of merging and disappearing into it, and, out of the blue, expressing the same fear about mother; or their difficulty staying in the room with me unless they could be near the door or the window, even with bars; or the person who has to be by the door of a plane at 10,000 feet in the air to avoid panic. As I have said, it is not only the mother but the early spatial structures constructed to replace the mother's internal space that are suffused with primitive emotional experiences.

As those spaces are structured by objects and their displacement, the objects in these spaces are gratifying or non-gratifying, persecuting or protecting, good or bad. Here are two dreams from two very schizoid patients. One dreamt that he was quite happy inside mother. He then felt he wanted to find out about outside, so he got out and started enjoying himself sexually and also doing aggressive things. He then became anxious as he felt some people might be angry with him, and that he was outside in the open and unprotected. So he got back inside mother. Unfortunately, he realized that it was not much safer because he could do things to his mother from inside that would put him in danger just the same.

Another schizoid young man dreamt that he was living in a sort of tunnel-like building and he was moving about in the tunnel in a sort of trolley. At intervals there were openings from which he could see the outside world. Sometimes the trolley would stop and he would get out to mix in with this outside world, especially for sexual purposes. Then he would get back and resume the inside life. However, one day he was seized with panic at the thought that the tunnel might close and he would be enclosed forever, and he desperately wanted to get out. There is nowhere for the claustro-agoraphobic.

An example of coming out of a containing space and something coming out of the body and their linking together by a common experience is given by the following patient, who was the most severe claustro-agoraphobic I have come across. He dreamt that he had passed a stool several hundred feet long which was still attached to his anus, unseparated from him. We proceeded with the session, and when the end of the session approached he sat on the couch in a state of extreme terror saying, 'Help me, help me. If I come out of the room, outside I will only be a mass of liquefied shit.'

Here we can see that coming out of the room was associated with faeces coming out of him, and the identification with the faeces was complete as he felt he would be nothing other than the faeces. Further, he could not in the dream let the faeces be separate from him. As he was himself identified with the faeces so he was afraid to be in open space, unprotected after he left me. This patient could only go to the lavatory to defecate if somebody knew he was in the toilet. He thus also demonstrates the fear of fragmentation if a part of him separates from the rest, and a fear of dissolution of self by identification with another object, such as the faeces.

It is obvious that problems of identity – for example, being small or adult, being male or female, and so on – are understandable on the above basis of transient identification with objects. Demandingness, controlling impulses, possessiveness are all clearly connected with the fact that the parts of the self-space put into the non-self-space and vice versa cannot be allowed separateness, and dictate such behaviour to prevent catastrophic loss of parts of the self. To prevent loss of self, objects must be kept at a distance and vice versa. Thus a young schizoid man in an attempt to solve this problem would remain in his room and communicate with others by watching children play from his window and communicating with others at a distance by telephone. A woman attempted to live in my personal space by constantly walking near my residence or using the telephone to penetrate into my flat. When there was nobody there she would let the telephone ring and fall asleep, being in my personal space. So the schizoid person, to prevent pain, anxiety or depression, splits parts of him or herself, projects them and denies their existence. Immediately he or she experiences the opposite feelings: fear of loss, of fragmentation, and attempts to remake contact, and the vicious circle goes on.

Internal and personal spaces are not the same. Personal-space objects are transitional between universal space and internal space. There is a story about Voltaire that describes how he built himself a tomb half in the church and half outside to confound those who argued about whether or not he was an atheist. The relative positioning of objects in space is astonishing at times. We know of the preoccupation of obsessions not to let objects touch each other, and the need for symmetry. But sometimes positioning is even more explicit. A very schizoid girl wondered if when objects were on top of each other, for example, a bird flying over her head, it meant sexual intercourse. After the death of her father she could not move because any movement would either hurt her father inside her or would have a sexual connotation. The relative positioning of objects was extremely meaningful to her.

She would put her right foot on top of the left and do a short, quick tapping movement. This was sexual, and was undone by putting the right foot from forwards to backwards, and instead of tapping she then did a larger and wider movement in the opposite direction.

I will now consider how immature 'concepts' of time are involved in a similar way of being. A little autistic boy who wanted his sessions at the same time every day, which I could not do, would take my watch and set it at the time he wanted. The time was the time indicated by the watch face, watches being very special spatial devices. We had to play a game of going from London to Brighton, and returning by train. We had to go from station to station and then return through each station in reverse order. Any fault on my part and everything had to be started all over again. He had seriated space as Piaget has demonstrated but could not decentre from it. He could pass from A to B to C to D, and so on, but not from D to A to return to A. He had to move from each position to the next like Achilles and the tortoise, or like Zeno's arrow. These examples lead us to examine more closely the elements of displacement and movement, and of time.

Piaget describes a simple experiment carried out with children of various ages. There are two tunnels, one visibly longer than the other. Two dolls, each on a separate track and moving at a fixed speed, are made to enter their respective tunnels at exactly the same time, and to emerge at the distal end also at exactly the same time. Children of a certain age repeatedly say the two dolls moved at the same speed, although they agree that one tunnel is longer. The tunnels are removed and the experiment repeated. This time, the same children will say that the doll overtaking the other one goes faster. However, if the tunnels are put back again, they say that the dolls were going at the same speed. They are clearly basing their judgement on the relative positioning of the dolls, irrespective of length and time. In that way, and by combining a large number of delightfully simple experiments, it is possible to reconstruct the stages through which the growing child passes as he constructs his adult ideas of space, speed, and time. At least these notions are involved in the notion of time: seriation or the ordering of events in time, for example, B comes after A, C after B, and so on; then class inclusion, for example, if B comes after A and C after B, then A-C is greater than A-B, or a whole class is greater than the subclass; finally, there is the measurement of time.

Similarly, the notion of causality is developed in stages and depends on the emergence of other notions such as those of the permanent object, of space and of time, leading to an objective view of causality instead of a magico-phenomenal one.

A woman, a very intelligent woman patient at that, said to me very seriously that she knows she will be married to me and live with me in my country of origin; that she will be married and live with her husband in England; and it will be the same with many other men – all simultaneously, without seeing any contradiction. In fact, she was angry at my suggesting there could be some difficulty in realizing this project.

'Time past is time future which is time present,' says T.S. Eliot (1944). But this is obviously time inconsistent. Time as a seriation process makes it impossible to go back in time. To be in the same place years later is not the same as previously. But displacement and movement to the schizoid can be disastrous, as it may tear part of him away and leave him fragmented or empty or lost, and it can do the same to his objects. Therefore, movements may be very slow or immobility may set in, as in the case of the girl with her father in her internal space. Movement brings about separation and loss, and if it comes fast, catastrophe. Rigidity, fixity, frigidity, impotence – are all defences against that possibility.

A very severely ill woman one day revealed to her therapist that she could not leave the hospital immediately after her session, which would be incompatible with her not collapsing. To take the bus and disappear quickly was dreadful. She wandered on the hospital ground first, and then very slowly moved away, very gradually. The speed at which she moved from one place to another mattered very much. In depression, movements of the body and limbs become slower and slower until a state of depressive stupor is reached; ultimate non-movement is found in suicide. In mania the contrary takes place: the speed of every movement including speed is increased and the patient cannot keep in one place. The sense of the passage of time is greatly altered in both states.

Piaget says:

> Psychological time is the connection between work accomplished and activity (force and rapidity of action) or time is plastic; it expands according to the deceleration or contracts according to the acceleration of action . . . or time is conferred at its point of departure with the impression of psychological duration inherent in the attitudes of expectations, effort, and of satisfaction in brief in the activity of the subject.
>
> (Battro 1973)

The schizoid patient, paralysed in his activities, empty of actions with objects, can only experience duration in relationships in a completely abnormal way.

It is necessary at this point to return to the relationship between localization of object and the most important notion of permanence of subject. Piaget describes frequently a little experiment showing how in the first half-year of mental life an infant who is about to grasp an object will stop his hands if the object is covered with a handkerchief. At a later stage the baby will try to lift the handkerchief to look for the object at the place A where it has just been covered. But, Piaget observes, if the object placed at A is displaced to B in front of the child watching the displacement, he will often look for the object at A, where he had been successful in finding it on previous occasions. It is only towards the end of the first year that the infant looks unhesitatingly for the object at the place to which it has been displaced; before this he ignores series of displacements, but is fixated on his own action on the object. Thus object permanence, says Piaget, is closely linked with its localization in space.

It is absolutely vital here to differentiate between the concept of object in Piaget and the libidinal object of psychoanalysis. Piaget describes an object as a permanent object at the end of the sensori-motor stage, at about eighteen months. Where the subject himself is an object among others, this concept applies to all objects and in no way considers the question of libidinal investment which renders an object meaningful and unique to the infant. The libidinal object is meaningful long before the completion of the sensori-motor object. Of vital interest for understanding distortions of self and object of the schizoid person are the stages of object formation described by Piaget, especially because of the specific use of objects of the physical world for identification purposes in schizoid mechanisms of defence.

Since the individual has also to construct his own body image as that of other bodies in space, and gradually to reach a sense of permanence of his identity, similar considerations apply here. As Marcel Proust (1982) has Swann say, if one wakes up in the night in the dark, not knowing the time or where one is, then one does not know who one is. It is extremely interesting that Piaget has demonstrated by lovely, simple little experiments that the concept of identity of matter takes place in definite stages, and that the concept of identity occurs, for instance, before the concept of conservation of quantity. Thus, by showing changing shapes of the same object, for instance, water, in differently shaped containers, it will take time before the child can say it is the same water. It will take more time before he is decentred from spatial ties such as believing there is more water in the tall thin tube than in the other. Only when able to co-ordinate two independent variables simultaneously, as width and height, will he achieve the right answer.

We now begin to understand the kind of level of organization of mental operations used by the schizoid patient when he feels instability, confusion of identity, disorder of body image, and fears of impermanence, since he is bound to experience himself differently in various localities, in various situations, with various objects.

The difficulty existing outside the space with which existence and permanence are so closely linked is enormous for the schizoid. Thus a young man only had a sense of existence when he drove his motor bike so long as there was a car in front of him or if his engine was going. If he passed the car or the engine stopped, he became depersonalized. A young woman, although she had changed greatly in analysis, could only be the person she was in her mother's head. A young man who lived alone for a considerable time in a room in a boarding house made progress, started studying, but had to move out of his room in order to have people about him, as he could not bear to be alone. So he sat in various public places like bars and cafés. Then he went through a phase when the place had to move with him, and so he sat on buses and wandered everywhere while studying. Was he being carried by mother everywhere? After months of this behaviour, he had a dream that he was standing in a bus holding a baby, his baby, and somewhat monstrous. Then the baby grew up and appeared normal, but he lost him. In his association he said the baby was also himself. Some phobics, and perhaps most, will go nowhere unless accompanied, and this can reach amazing extremes with some patients.

For this paper I have attempted to introduce concepts of space, movement and time as the basic elements, the weft and warp of primitive human behaviour. Primitive thought is centred on the first moves taken by the infant to structure space. This is done by the action of the subject on his objects and vice versa. Primitive notions of time then follow. Patterns of behaviour belonging to any stage may persist and become active at any time later.

References

Battro, M. (1973). *Piaget: A Dictionary of Terms* (E. Ritschverimann and S.F. Cambell, Eds). Pergamon.

Bion, W.R. (1965). Transformations. In *Seven Servants: Four Works*. Jason Aronson.

Eliot, T.S. (1944). *Four Quartets*. Faber and Faber.

Freud, S. (1909). Notes Upon a Case of Obsessional Neurosis. In *SE* (Vol. 10). Hogarth, 1953–1974.

Guntrip, H. (1968). *Schizoid Phenomena, Object Relations and the Self*. Hogarth.

Laplanche, J., and Pontalis, J.B. (1973). *The Language of Psycho-Analysis* (D. Nicholson-Smith, Trans.). Norton.

Proust, M. (1982). *Remembrance of Things Past* (C.K. Scott Moncrieff and T. Kilmartin, Trans.). Vintage Press.

Rey, H. (1994). The Schizoid Mode of Being and the Space-Time Continuum (Before Metaphor). In J. Magnana (Ed.), *Universals of Psychoanalysis in the Treatment of Psychotic and Borderline States*. Free Association Books.

Rey, J.H. (1988). That Which Patients Bring to Analysis. *International Journal of Psychoanalysis*. 69:457–470.

Steiner, J. (1994). *Psychic Retreats: Pathological Organizations in Psychotic, Neurotic and Borderline Patients*. Routledge.

Chapter 8

A Theory of Psychic Retreats

John Steiner

SUMMARY

John Steiner collaborated with Henri Rey at the Maudsley Hospital and developed an interest in highly complex organizations, which he named psychic retreats. Clinically, they manifested themselves in dead ends and stuck situations where the patient seems difficult to reach. The analyst feels that his efforts remain futile since the patient seems to maintain a precarious psychic equilibrium, which protects him from anxiety, guilt, and pain but also obstructs psychic development and change. Theoretically, those 'pathological organizations of the personality', as Steiner describes them, can be thought of either as a combination of various defensive mechanisms or as a network of object relations. Steiner localizes them at the border between the paranoid-schizoid and depressive positions, which he called the 'borderline position'. His clear description of those organizations has largely influenced the development of psychoanalytic theory and technique. The paper reprinted in this volume is the introductory chapter to his book *Psychic Retreats* (Steiner 1993).

Patients who live under the grip of a pathological organization lack emotional contact and clearly display features of the claustro-agoraphobic dilemma: they can reside neither inside nor outside their objects. As Steiner emphasizes, psychic retreats may be represented in an interpersonal form as a sect, a business organization, a mafia-like gang, or in a spatial form such as a hiding place, a cave, a safe haven, a desert island, or a prison. It is particularly the spatial representation that shows, together with the timelessness, the characteristics of the claustro-agoraphobic situation. Steiner's theory can be seen as an extension and further evolution of Melanie Klein's, Hanna Segal's, Herbert Rosenfeld's, and Henri Rey's ideas. It also offers new insight into the problem of how to reach those patients who are caught in such desperate places and often are addictively dependent on the false promises the psychic retreat offers them.

TEXT

A psychic retreat provides the patient with an area of relative peace and protection from strain when meaningful contact with the analyst is experienced as threatening.

DOI: 10.4324/9781003200284-8

It is not difficult to understand the need for transient withdrawal of this kind, but serious technical problems arise in patients who turn to a psychic retreat, habitually, excessively, and indiscriminately. In some analyses, particularly with borderline and psychotic patients, a more or less permanent residence in the retreat may be taken up and it is then that obstacles to development and growth arise.

In my own clinical experience this type of withdrawal and the resultant failure to allow contact with the analyst takes many forms. An aloof type of schizoid superiority is expressed as a cold condescension in one patient and as a mocking dismissal of my work in another. Some patients are clearly reacting to anxiety, and their withdrawal appears to indicate that the analysis has touched on a sensitive topic which has to be avoided. Perhaps the most difficult type of retreat is that in which a false type of contact is offered and the analyst is invited to engage in ways which seem superficial, dishonest, or perverse. Sometimes these reactions can be seen to result from clumsy or intrusive behaviour on the part of the analyst, but it often happens that even careful analysis leaves the patients out of contact. They retreat behind a powerful system of defences which serve as a protective armour or hiding place, and it is sometimes possible to observe how they emerge with great caution like a snail coming out of its shell and retreat once more if contact leads to pain or anxiety.

We have come to understand that obstacles to contact and obstacles to progress and development are related, and that they both arise from the deployment of a particular type of defensive organization by means of which the patient hopes to avoid intolerable anxiety. I call such systems of defences *'pathological organizations of the personality'* and use this term to denote a family of defensive systems which are characterized by extremely unyielding defences and which function to help the patient to avoid anxiety by avoiding contact with other people and with reality. The pursuit of this approach has led me to examine in more detail the way defences operate and, in particular, how they interconnect to form complex, closely knit defensive systems.

The analyst observes psychic retreats as states of mind in which the patient is stuck, cut off, and out of reach, and he may infer that these states arise from the operation of a powerful system of defences. The patient's view of the retreat is reflected in the descriptions which he gives and also in unconscious phantasy as it is revealed in dreams, memories, and reports from everyday life which give a pictorial or dramatized image of how the retreat is unconsciously experienced. Typically it appears as a house, a cave, a fortress, a desert island, or a similar location which is seen as an area of relative safety. Alternatively, it can take an interpersonal form, usually as an organization of objects or part-objects which offers to provide security. It may be represented as a business organization, as a boarding school, as a religious sect, as a totalitarian government or a Mafia-like gang. Often tyrannical and perverse elements are evident in the description, but sometimes the organization is idealized and admired.

Usually over a period of time various representations can be observed which help to build up a picture of the patient's defensive organization. Later I will try to show that it is sometimes useful to think of it as a grouping of object relations, defences, and phantasies which makes up a borderline position similar to but distinct from the paranoid-schizoid and the depressive positions described by Melanie Klein (1952).

The relief provided by the retreat is achieved at the cost of isolation, stagnation, and withdrawal, and some patients find such a state distressing and complain about it. Others, however, accept the situation with resignation, relief, and at times defiance or triumph, so that it is the analyst who has to cany the despair associated with the failure to make contact. Sometimes the retreat is experienced as a cruel place and the deadly nature of the situation is recognized by the patient, but more often the retreat is idealized and represented as a pleasant and even ideal haven. Whether idealized or persecutory, it is clung to as preferable to even worse states which the patient is convinced are the only alternatives. In most patients some movement is observable as they cautiously emerge from the retreat only to return again when things go wrong. In some cases true development is possible in these periods of emergence, and the patient is gradually able to lessen his propensity to withdraw.

In others withdrawal is more prolonged, and if emergence does take place the gains achieved are transitory and the patient returns to his previous state in a negative therapeutic reaction. Typically, an equilibrium is reached in which the patient uses the retreat to remain relatively free from anxiety but at the cost of an almost complete standstill in development. The situation is complicated by the fact that the analyst is used as part of the defensive organization and is sometimes so subtly invited to join in that he does not realize that the analysis itself has been converted into a retreat. The analyst is often under great pressure, and his frustration may lead him to despair or to mount a usually futile effort to overcome what are perceived as the patient's stubborn defences. All gradations of dependence on the retreat are found clinically, from the completely stuck patient at one extreme to those who use the retreat in a transient and discretionary way at the other. The range and pervasiveness of the retreat may also vary, and some patients are able to develop and sustain adequate relationships in some areas but remain stuck in other aspects of their lives. One of the points I will emphasize throughout this book is that change is possible even in the analysis of very stuck patients. If the analyst is able to persevere and survive the pressure he is put under, he and the patient can gradually come to gain some insight into the operation of the organization and to loosen the grip and the range of its operation.

One of the features of the retreat which emerges most clearly in perverse, psychotic, and borderline patients is the way the avoidance of contact with the analyst is at the same time an avoidance of contact with reality. The retreat then serves as an area of the mind where reality does not have to be faced, where phantasy and omnipotence can exist unchecked and where anything is permitted. This feature is often what makes the retreat so attractive to the patient and commonly involves the use of perverse or psychotic mechanisms.

I am impressed by the power of the system of defences which one can observe operating in these stuck analyses. Sometimes they are so successful that the patient is protected from anxiety, and no difficulty arises as long as the system remains unchallenged. Others remain stuck in the retreat despite the evident suffering it brings, which may be chronic and sustained or masochistic and addictive. In all of these, however, the patient is threatened by the possibility of change and, if provoked, may respond with a more profound withdrawal.

These situations are of great theoretical interest but my own concern is primarily clinical, and this means that my central preoccupation is with the way organizations function in individual patients in individual sessions during an analysis. Here it is important to recognize that the analyst is never able to be an uninvolved observer since he is always to a greater or lesser degree enlisted to participate in enactments in the transference (Sandler 1976; Sandler and Sandler 1978; Joseph 1989). In developing these ideas in the area of pathological organizations I have taken note of the way the patient will use the analyst to help create a sanctuary into which he can retreat. I have been most concerned to follow the situation in the fine grain of the session and to describe how the patient makes moves to emerge from the sanctuary only to retreat again when he confronts anxieties he cannot or will not bear.

It was the highly organized nature of the process which struck me and which led me to use the term 'pathological organization' to describe the internal configuration of defences. The clinical picture itself has become familiar to most working analysts and has been described in various terms by a number of writers whose work is reviewed later in the book. Abraham's (1919, 1924) study of narcissistic resistance and Reich's (1933) work on 'character armour' are early examples. Riviere (1936) spoke about a highly organized system of defences, and Rosenfeld (1964, 1971) described the operation of destructive narcissism. Segal (1972), O'Shaughnessy (1981), Riesenberg-Malcolm (1981), and Joseph (1982, 1983) have also described patients caught up in powerful defensive systems. This and other similar work has been concerned with patients in extreme situations which can be thought of in relation to those ultimate obstacles to change which Freud addressed in 'Analysis terminable and interminable' (1937). Freud linked these deepest obstacles to change to the operation of the death instinct and, in my view, pathological organizations have a particular role to play in the universal problem of dealing with primitive destructiveness. This affects the individual in profound ways, whether it arises from external or internal sources. Traumatic experiences with violence or neglect in the environment leads to the internalization of violent disturbed objects which at the same time serve as suitable receptacles for the projection of the individual's own destructiveness.

It is not necessary to resolve controversial issues about the death instinct to recognize that there is often something very deadly and self-destructive in the individual's make-up which threatens his integrity unless it is adequately contained. In my view, defensive organizations serve to bind, to neutralize, and to control primitive destructiveness whatever its source, and are a universal feature of the defensive make-up of all individuals. Moreover, in some patients where problems related to destructiveness are particularly prominent, the organization comes to dominate the psyche, and it is these cases which allow its mode of operation to be most readily appreciated. Once recognized, similar if less disturbing versions can be identified in neurotic and normal individuals.

It is not clear if these methods of dealing with the destructiveness are ever really successful. Certainly, the forms of organization we usually observe tend to function as a kind of compromise and are as much an expression of the destructiveness as a defence against it. Because of this compromise they are always pathological, even though they may serve an adaptive purpose and provide an area of relief and transient protection. Pathological organizations stultify the personality, prevent contact with reality, and ensure that growth and development are interfered with. In normal individuals they are brought into play when anxiety exceeds tolerable limits and are relinquished once more when the crisis is over. Nevertheless, they remain potentially available and can serve to take the patient out of contact and give rise to a stuck period of analysis if the analytic work touches on issues at the edge of what is tolerable. In the more disturbed patient they come to dominate the personality and the patient is to a greater or lesser degree caught in their grip.

The distinction between psychotic and non-psychotic parts of the personality introduced by Bion (1957) can help to differentiate the types of organization which arise in severely disturbed patients from those which exist in neurotic and normal patients, and this is discussed in a chapter, where a psychotic organization is described. In psychotic and borderline patients, the organization dominates the personality, where it is used to patch up damaged parts of the ego and as a result is indispensable to the psychotic part of the personality. The non-psychotic personality is less likely to make destructive attacks on its own mind, and since the situation is less desperate a more fluid type of alternation between projective and introjective processes can occur. Despite these differences there are many elements which pathological organizations of the personality in different types of patients have in common and which come to the fore when the patient is under pressure. If analytic work attempts to help the patient deal with problems at the limit of his capacity, difficult areas are raised even in patients who normally function relatively well, and in these situations the patient is likely to make use of a retreat to which he may in normal circumstances only rarely resort. Even in normal and neurotic patients when the retreat is often represented as a space which occurs naturally or is provided by the environment, it can be seen to arise from the operation of powerful systems of defences. Occasionally patients themselves recognize how they create the retreat, and may even be able to identify the way it serves as a defence.

Mostly, however, the description in terms of defences represents the analyst's point of view and forms part of the analyst's theoretical approach. I have found a close examination of the object relations as they emerge in the transference to be particularly helpful in revealing some of the basic mechanisms which are involved in the workings of a pathological organization. To understand the details of their structure it is necessary to know something about the operation of primitive mechanisms of defence, and in particular about projective identification, which is such a central concept in modern Kleinian psychoanalysis. These are discussed later in the book, and at this point it will suffice to recognize that projective identification leads to a narcissistic type of object relationship similar to that which Freud described perhaps most clearly in his paper on Leonardo (1910). In the most straightforward type of projective identification a part of the self is split off and projected into an object, where it is attributed to the object and the fact that it belongs to the self is denied. The object relationship which results is then not with a person truly seen as separate, but with the self projected into another person and related to as if it were someone else. This is the position of the mythical Narcissus, who fell in love with a strange youth he did not consciously connect with himself. It is also true of Leonardo, who projected his infantile self into his apprentices and looked after them in the way he wished his mother had looked after him (Freud 1910).

A narcissistic type of object relationship based on projective identification is certainly a central aspect of pathological organizations, but this is not in itself sufficient to explain the enormous power and resistance to change which they demonstrate. Moreover, projective identification is not in itself a pathological mechanism and indeed forms the basis of all empathic communication. We project into others to understand better what it feels like to be in their shoes, and an inability or reluctance to do this profoundly affects object relations. However, it is essential to normal mental function to be able to use projective identification in a flexible and reversible way and thus to be able to withdraw projections and to observe and interact with others from a position firmly based in our own identity.

In many pathological states such reversibility is obstructed and the patient is unable to regain parts of the self lost through projective identification, and consequently loses touch with aspects of his personality which permanently reside in objects with whom they become identified. Any attribute such as intelligence, warmth, masculinity, aggression, and so on can be projected and disowned in this way and, when reversibility is blocked, results in a depletion of the ego no longer has access to the lost parts of the self. At the same time, the object is distorted by having attributed to it the split-off and denied parts of the self.

The study of pathological organizations reported in this book has led me to postulate further complexities of structure. The kind of defensive situation just outlined can arise as a result of normal splitting in which the object is seen as either good or bad and the individual tries to get the help of the good to protect him from the bad. It is clear, as Klein herself emphasized (1952), that such splitting of the object is always accompanied by a corresponding split in the ego, and it is a good part of the self in a relationship with a good object which is kept separate from a bad part of the self in relation to a bad object. If the split is successfully maintained, the good and bad are kept so separate that no interaction between them takes place, but if it threatens to break down, the individual may try to preserve his equilibrium by turning to the protection of the good object and good parts of the self against the bad object and against bad parts of the self. If such measures also fail to maintain an equilibrium, even more drastic means may be resorted to. For example, pathological splitting with a fragmentation of the self and of the object and their expulsion in a more violent and primitive form of projective identification may take place (Bion 1957). Pathological organizations may then evolve to collect the fragments, and the result may once again give the impression of a protective good object kept separate from bad ones. Now, however, what appears as a relatively straightforward split between good and bad is in fact the result of a splitting of the personality into several elements, each projected into objects and reassembled in a manner which simulates the containing function of an object. The organization may present itself as a good object protecting the individual from destructive attacks, but in fact its structure is made up of good and bad elements derived from the self and from the objects which have been projected into and used as building blocks for the resultant extremely complex organization. In my view, the dependent self which is dominated by the organization may also be complex and not as innocent a victim as may first appear. It is not only the building blocks of the organization which need to be understood but the manner in which they are assembled and held together, because the dependent part of the self, and the analyst too, may become caught up and trapped in the tyrannical and cruel object relations which keep the system intact.

In later chapters I will try to show how in pathological organizations of the personality projective identification is not confined to a single object, but, instead, groups of objects are used which are themselves in a relationship. These objects, usually in fact part-objects, are constructed out of experiences with people found in the patient's early environment. The fantastic figures of the patient's inner world are sometimes based on actual experiences with bad objects and sometimes represent distortions and misrepresentations of early experience. Trauma and deprivation in the patient's history have a profound effect on the creation of pathological organizations of the personality, even though it may not be possible to know how much internal and external factors contributed. What becomes apparent in the here and now of the analysis is that the objects, whether they are chosen from those which pre-exist in the environment or created by the individual, are used for specific defensive purposes, in particular to bind destructive elements in the personality. I have argued that a central function of pathological organizations of the personality is to contain and neutralize these primitive destructive impulses, and in order to deal with these the patient selects destructive objects into which he can project destructive parts of the self. As Rosenfeld (1971), Meltzer (1968) and others have described, these objects are often assembled into a 'gang' which is held together by cruel and violent means. These powerfully structured groups of individuals are represented unconsciously in the patient's inner world and appear in dreams as an inter-personal version of the retreat. The place of safety is provided by the group who offer protection from both persecution and guilt as long as the patient does not threaten the domination of the gang. The result of these operations is to create a complex network of object relations, each object containing split-off parts of the self and the group held together in complex ways characteristic of a particular organization. The organization 'contains' the anxiety by offering itself as a protector, and it does so in a perverse way very different from that seen in the case of normal containment, such as that described by Bion, to take place between a normal mother and her baby (Bion 1962, 1963). This formulation illustrates the extent to which the organization can become personified. In part this is a result of its evolution in early infancy, when many aspects of nature are experienced by the child as arising from the actions of people. In part, however, it results from the way the inner world remains one peopled by objects in relationships with each other as well as with the subject. No sanctuary is secure unless it is also sanctioned and protected by the social group to which it belongs. Sometimes it is possible to get information about deeper phantasies in which psychic retreats appear as spaces inside objects or part-objects. There may be phantasies of retreating to the mother's womb, anus, or breast, sometimes experienced as a desirable but forbidden place.

One of the major consequences of such a structure is that it is very difficult for the individual to risk a confrontation with these objects and repudiate their methods and aims. As a result, the reversibility of projective identification is interfered with. I will argue later that this reversibility is established through a successful working through of mourning. The process of regaining parts of the self lost through projective identification involves facing the reality of what belongs to the object and what belongs to the self, and this is established most clearly through the experience of loss. It is in the process of mourning that parts of the self are regained, and this achievement may require much working through. Thus a true internalization of the object can only be achieved if it is relinquished as an external object. It can then be internalized as separate from the self and in this state can be identified with in a flexible and reversible way. The development of symbolic function assists this process and allows the individual to identify with aspects of the object rather than its concrete totality.

When containment is provided by an organization of objects rather than by a single object it is very difficult for projective identification to be reversed. It is not possible to let any single object go, mourn it, and, in the process, withdraw projections from it, because it does not operate in isolation but has powerful links which bind it to other members of the organization. These links are often ruthlessly maintained, with the primary aim of keeping the organization intact. In fact, the individuals are often experienced as bound inextricably to each other and the containment is felt to be provided by a group of objects treated as if it were a single object; namely, the organization.

To withdraw projections from one of the objects means that reality has to be faced in the area of that particular object relationship and then what belongs to the object and what belongs to the self must be differentiated so that the projection can be separated off and returned to the self. Even if defences operate singly this may be difficult, but when the object relations are part of a complex organization the inter-relationships ensure that the difficulty is extreme. The patient then feels trapped in an omnipotent organization from which there is no escape. If the analyst recognizes the omnipotence he or she is less likely to try to confront or combat the organization head-on. Such recognition, in my view, helps both analyst and patient to live with the omnipotence without either giving in to it or aggressively confronting it. If it can be recognized as one of the facts of life making up the reality of the patient's inner world, then gradually it may become possible to understand it better and as a result to reduce the hold it has on the personality.

I have emphasized how pathological organizations of the personality can result in a stuck patient in a stuck analysis, who may be so hidden from contact that it is difficult for the analyst to reach him. In other patients a similar overall situation results not so much from the lack of contact, movement, and development as from the fact that any development which does occur is quickly, and sometimes totally, reversed. Once this is recognized it is often possible to see that similar, more subtle movements are discernible even in the most apparently stuck patient. As a result a more detailed description becomes possible, which involves following the patient as he makes tentative, sometimes almost imperceptible, moves towards contact with the analyst, only to retreat once more as he confronts anxiety. As the patient begins to emerge from the protection of the organization the ready availability of the shelter as a source of relief of anxiety and pain makes retreat a convenient option, and sometimes the experience of contact is so dreaded that withdrawal is immediate. Nevertheless, if this moment of contact is registered by the analyst and interpreted, the patient can sometimes gain an insight into his dread of contact, feel supported by the analyst, and as a result may gradually extend his ability to tolerate it.

If the patient feels the analyst understands the nature of the anxieties which confront him as he begins to emerge from his retreat, he is more likely to feel supported and thus take further steps away from his dependence on the pathological organization of the personality. Here an important distinction exists between the anxieties of the paranoid-schizoid and those of the depressive positions as described by Klein (1946, 1952), and pathological organizations of the personality serve to protect the patient against both sets of anxieties (Steiner 1979, 1987). This point of view suggests that it is important not only to describe the mental mechanisms which operate at any particular moment but also to discuss their function: that is, not only what is happening but why it is happening – in this instance to try to understand what it is that the patient fears would result if he emerged from the retreat. If the minute movements are attended to, a transient and briefly bearable 'taste' of the anxiety which is experienced on emergence from the retreat can be registered by the patient and interpreted by the analyst as it becomes observable. This can allow the function of the defence to be identified and investigated. Some patients depend on the organization to protect them from primitive states of fragmentation and persecution, and they fear that states of extreme anxiety would overwhelm them if they were to emerge from the retreat. Others have been able to develop a greater degree of integration but are unable to face the depressive pain and guilt which arise as contact with internal and external reality increases. In either case, emergence to make contact with the analyst may lead to a rapid withdrawal to the retreat and an attempt to regain the previously held equilibrium.

Melanie Klein (1952) described the paranoid-schizoid and depressive positions in terms of a grouping of defences, and a pattern of anxieties and other emotions. Each is characterized also by typical mental structures and by typical forms of object relationship, both internal and external. It is in relationship to these positions that pathological organizations can most readily be understood, and indeed the retreat can also be thought of as a position with its own grouping of anxieties, its pattern of defences, its typical object relations and characteristic structure. I have previously referred to it as a borderline position' because of its place on the border between the two basic positions (Steiner 1987, 1990).

The terminology of the positions can be confusing because of the inferred connection to particular types of clinical disorder. Klein had to emphasize that the paranoid-schizoid position did not imply paranoid psychosis in any simple way nor the depressive position, depressive illness. In the same way, the term 'borderline position' is not confined to borderline patients, and although it is true that psychic retreats can be readily observed in borderline states they are also a prominent feature of psychotic patients at one extreme and of normal and neurotic individuals at times of stress, at the other. Klein herself occasionally spoke of a manic position and an obsessional position (Klein 1946), and these more organized defensive states have many features in common with psychic retreats. It is clear that not only the basic two positions but also the borderline position occur in all patients, and the notion of positions can help the analyst to consider where the patient is located at any particular time.

The patient can withdraw to a retreat at a borderline position where he is under the protection of a pathological organization from either of the two basic positions. This theme is elaborated later in the book, where use is made of a triangular equilibrium diagram to illustrate that as the patient emerges from the retreat he may find himself confronted with anxieties from either of the two basic positions.

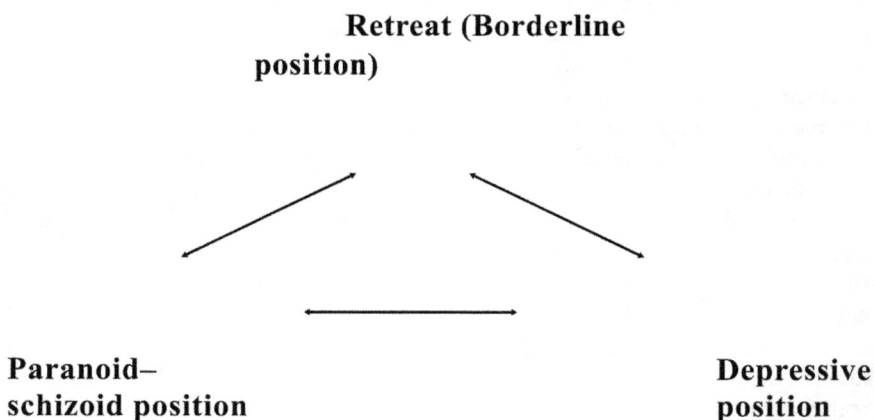

Retreat (Borderline position)

Paranoid– schizoid position

Depressive position

Figure 8.1 Triad of equilibrium.

When the analysis is stuck there is very little, if any, movement discernible in this equilibrium, and the patient becomes firmly established in the retreat protected by the pathological organization and only rarely emerges to face either depressive or paranoid-schizoid anxieties. In less stuck situations, which of course occur in patients who may nevertheless be quite ill, and even psychotic, more movement is discernible and shifts occur in which anxieties are at least transiently faced. Here the loss of equilibrium may give rise to severe anxiety and immediate return to the retreat, but it may also enable analytic development to take place.

A striking finding with some examples of a pathological organization of the personality is that the organization is adhered to even when some development has taken place and the need for it no longer appears to be so convincing. It is as if the patient has become accustomed and even addicted to the state of affairs in the retreat and gains a kind of perverse gratification from it. The part of the patient which is in touch with reality is often seduced away by bribes and threats, and the whole organization keeps itself together by creating perverse links between its component members. Indeed, perverse mechanisms play a central role in pathological organizations, particularly in cementing the organization together and underpinning its immovable structure.

A particular type of relationship with reality which is characteristic of retreats plays an important role in preventing the move towards the depressive position which is necessary for development to occur. Freud, in his discussion of fetishism (Freud 1927), described how the patient adopts a stance in which reality is neither fully accepted nor fully disavowed, so that contradictory views are held simultaneously and are reconciled in a variety of ways. In my view, a central aspect of the perverse attitude is reflected in this kind of relation to reality. It is important in *sexual* perversions, where some of the basic 'facts of life', such as the difference between the sexes and between the generations, are simultaneously accepted and disavowed, but it has a more general applicability to any aspect of reality which is difficult to accept. In particular, we see it prominent in the difficult task of facing the reality of ageing and death to which a similarly perverse stance is often taken. A perverse pseudo-acceptance of reality is one of the factors which makes the retreat so attractive for the patient who can keep sufficient contact with reality to appear 'normal' while at the same time evading its most painful aspects.

A second aspect of perversion is seen when the object relations which make up the organization are examined. The links which bind the organization together are often sado-masochistic and involve a cruel type of tyranny in which objects and the patient himself are controlled and bullied in a ruthless way. Sometimes the sadism is obvious, but often the tyranny is idealized and develops a seductive hold on the patient, who appears to become addicted to it, often gaining a masochistic gratification in the process.

It is only with long and painful work that the patient begins to feel he has the capacity to say 'no' to the attractive pull of the perversion as alternative sources of help become available. He may then feel less entrapped by the organization and feel he only need turn to its protection at times of particular stress. As the addictive properties lessen he is able to free himself more and face psychic reality. Once this becomes even partially possible, mourning and loss lead to a partial recovery of parts of the self and the dependence on the organization is further loosened. It nevertheless always remains part of the personality where the patient can retreat when reality becomes unbearable. If it is recognized for what it is – namely, an area where perverse relationships and perverse thinking are sanctioned – the patient may accept an occasional need to adopt these methods without idealizing them. The protection of the retreat is then seen to offer a temporary respite from anxiety but no real security and no opportunity for development. Like other elements in the inner world, it can then be viewed more realistically and the patient can come to terms with it.

This preliminary outline will be expanded in the following chapters. It is clear that a psychic retreat can be conceptualized in a variety of different ways. First, it can be viewed spatially as an area of safety to which the patient withdraws, and second, this area can be seen to depend on the operation of a pathological organization of the personality. The organization itself can be seen as a highly structured system of defences and also as a tightly organized network of object relations. The retreat may also be usefully related to the paranoid-schizoid and depressive positions and can then be seen to function as a third position to which the patient can withdraw from the anxieties of either of the former. Finally, the perverse nature of the retreat can be viewed from the point of view of the patient's relationship with reality on the one hand and in terms of the sadomasochistic type of object relationships found, on the other.

Patients who find themselves trapped in a psychic retreat present formidable technical problems for the analyst. He has to struggle to cope with a patient who is out of contact and an analysis which seems to be getting nowhere for very long periods. The analyst also has to struggle with his own propensity both to fit in and collude with the organization on the one hand and to withdraw into his own defensive retreat, on the other. If the analyst comes to understand some of the processes better, he is more able to recognize the patient's situation and to be available at those times when the patient does emerge to make contact possible.

References

Abraham, K. (1919). A Particular Form of Neurotic Resistance against the Psychoanalytic Method. In *Selected Papers of Karl Abraham* (pp. 303–311). Hogarth Press.

Abraham, K. (1924). A Short Study of the Development of the Libido, Viewed in the Light of Mental Disorders. In *Selected Papers of Karl Abraham* (pp. 418–501). Hogarth Press.

Bion, W.R. (1957). Differentiation of the Psychotic from the Non-Psychotic Personalities. *International Journal of Psychoanalysis*, *38*, 266–275.

Bion, W.R. (1962). *Learning from Experience*. Heinemann.

Bion, W.R. (1963). *Elements of Psycho-Analysis*. Heinemann.

Freud, S. (1910). Leonardo Da Vinci and a Memory of His Childhood. In *SE* (Vol. 11, pp. 63–137).

Freud, S. (1927). Fetishis. In *SE* (Vol. 21, pp. 152–157).

Freud, S. (1937). Analysis Terminable and Interminable. In *SE* (Vol. 23, pp. 216–253).

Joseph, B. (1982). Addiction to Near Death. *International Journal of Psychoanalysis*, *63*, 449–456.

Joseph, B. (1983). On Understanding and Not Understanding: Some Technical Issues. *International Journal of Psychoanalysis*, *64*, 291–298.

Joseph, B. (1989). *Psychic Equilibrium and Psychic Change: Selected Papers of Betty Joseph* (M. Feldman and E. Bott Spillius, Eds). Routledge.

Klein, M. (1946). Notes on Some Schizoid Mechanisms. *International Journal of Psychoanalysis*, *27*, 99–110.

Klein, M. (1952). Some Theoretical Conclusions Regarding the Emotional Life of the Infant. In J. Riviere (Ed.), *Developments in Psychoanalysis*. Hogarth Press.

Meltzer, D. (1968). Terror, Persecution, Dread. *International Journal of Psychoanalysis*, *49*, 396–401.

O'Shaughnessy, E. (1981). A Clinical Study of a Defensive Organization. *International Journal of Psychoanalysis*, *62*, 359–369.

Reich, W. (1933). *Character Analysis*. Orgone Institute Press.

Riesenberg-Malcolm, R. (1981). Expiation as a Defence. *International Journal of Psychoanalytic Psychotherapy*, *8*, 549–570.

Riviere, J. (1936). A Contribution to the Analysis of the Negative Therapeutic Reaction. *International Journal of Psychoanalysis*, *17*, 304–320.

Rosenfeld, H.A. (1964). On the Psychopathology of Narcissism: A Clinical Approach. *International Journal of Psychoanalysis*, *45*, 332–337.

Rosenfeld, H.A. (1971). A Clinical Approach to the Psychoanalytic Theory of the Life and Death Instincts: An Investigation into the Aggressive Aspects of Narcissism. *International Journal of Psychoanalysis*, *52*, 169–178.

Sandler, J. (1976). Countertransference and Role-responsiveness. *International Review of Psycho-Analysis*, *3*, 43–47.

Sandler, J., and Sandler, A.M. (1978). On the Development of Object Relationships and Affects. *International Journal of Psychoanalysis*, *59*, 285–296.

Segal, H. (1972). A Delusional System as a Defence Against the Re-emergence of a Catastrophic Situation. *International Journal of Psychoanalysis*, *53*, 393–401.

Steiner, J. (1979). The Border between the Paranoid-Schizoid and the Depressive Positions in the Borderline Patient. *British Journal of Medical Psychology*, *52*, 385–391.

Steiner, J. (1987). The Interplay between Pathological Organisations and the Paranoid-Schizoid and Depressive Positions. *International Journal of Psychoanalysis*, *68*, 69–80.

Steiner, J. (1990). Pathological Organisations as Obstacles to Mourning: The Role of Unbearable Guilt. *International Journal of Psychoanalysis*, *71*, 87–94.

Steiner, J. (1993). *Psychic Retreats: Pathological Organizations in Psychotic, Neurotic and Borderline Patients*. Routledge.

Chapter 9

Monstrous Phantasies and Monstrous Gods

Claustro-Agoraphobic Anxiety in Hesiod and Klein

Susan Finkelstein

SUMMARY

In her work with young children, Melanie Klein observed monstrous uncon-scious phantasies and claustro-agoraphobic anxieties that the Greek poet Hesiod described 2,700 years earlier in his epic poem *Theogony*, the genealogy of the gods. Claustrophobic fears of imprisonment within the mother's body and agora-phobic wishes to return to the womb, alongside the fear of being shut out of it, are terrifying themes found in mythology and universal truths of humankind. They are the recurrent beliefs and fears of small children and adults found in Greek mythology, fairy tales, and psychoanalysis. Whereas Freud developed the Oedi-pus complex from the writings of Sophocles, Klein postulated an earlier, maternal version of the Oedipus complex. "Monstrous Phantasies and Monstrous Gods" links the work of Hesiod with that of the psychoanalyst Melanie Klein. This paper addresses some important correspondences between Hesiod and Klein as their vision pertains to the claustro-agoraphobic dilemma and the acceptance of reality, guilt, and reparation as defined by Henri Rey.

TEXT

Children are noticing and inquisitive creatures. So are psychoanalysts and poets. It was Sophocles, after all, from whom Freud borrowed the Oedipus complex, and Sophocles had a predecessor, Hesiod, who had begun exploring the border between myth and psychology four centuries earlier, circa 800 BC. Hesiod and his contemporary Homer are the oldest known writers in the western literary tradition, and Hesiod's *Theogony* is one of its first documented works. In it, Hesiod took the earliest questions – "Who am I?" and "Where did I come from?" – and elabo-rated them in an extravagantly detailed mythology of sexuality, reproduction, and parent-child relationship. The power and clarity of his vision are apparent in the *Theogony*'s endurance as a work of literature and in its uncanny resemblance to phantasies that we see in our children, our patients, and often, when we are paying attention, ourselves.

DOI: 10.4324/9781003200284-9

Freud's debt to Sophocles is well established, but Hesiod's tales of sadism, violence, omnipotence, and complex maternal oedipal figures resonate with Melanie Klein's descriptions of the unconscious mental life of infants and children.

Klein is distinctive among analysts for the stunning explicitness of the phantasies she attributed to very young children. She first observed them in her patients but eventually understood them to be universal conclusions about sexual life as people at characteristic stages of their psychic development come to apprehend it.

As Freud thought that dreams (and associations with them) were the royal road to the unconscious, Klein felt that the storytelling of children was the key to their private mental lives and one of their chief ways of dealing with anxiety, conflict, and sexual discovery. In particular, she recognized in children's stories the hidden secrets and fears and the resulting annihilation anxieties that arise from their dawning awareness of sexuality and the drama of the primal couple. Especially in a therapeutic setting, she thought, children invent characters, identify with them, and tell stories about them, "personifying" them to represent their parents, their siblings, and their internal world of objects (1929, p. 199). She did not hesitate to interpret these personifications or their transferential meanings, both positive and negative.

The stories that Klein heard in this way mirror startlingly the ones told by Hesiod, which came down to him through generations of oral tradition and which clearly had been haunting the human race for thousands of years before Klein discovered them in her young patients. Let me state explicitly here that I do not assume that Klein had knowledge of Hesiod's work. Nor do I imply that she did not arrive at her conclusions independently, exactly as she recounts. But there are striking and illuminating parallels between her work and his, despite the vast gulf of time between them and the inevitable differences between a literary act and a scientific one, and it is time to recognize them. In "Some Reflections on the *Oresteia*" Klein states,

> The fear of such punishment goes back to the fact that greed and envy are first of all experienced toward the mother who is felt to be injured by these emotions and who by projection turns in the child's mind into a greedy and resentful figure. She is therefore feared as a source of punishment, the prototype of God.
>
> (p. 280)

In this study, therefore, I will explore Hesiod's great creation epic *Theogony* (that is, *the genealogy of the gods)* to provide an expanded cultural context for Klein's work and to outline some of the larger implications of her clinical intuition. In essence, Hesiod's depiction of the origins of the gods and the human race is a family myth, such as psychoanalysts encounter in dream representations and other unconscious phantasies. My intention for now is simply to demonstrate some of the more important overlaps between Hesiod's vision and Klein's, in particular as they pertain to one of my enduring interests – what Henri Rey (1994, p. 9) called the *claustro-agoraphobic syndrome*, about which more shortly. If nothing else, this exercise makes clear that the phantasies that Klein attributes universally to human beings (which are disconcerting and often fiercely resisted even within the psychoanalytic community) were widespread in ancient Greece; it, therefore, offers support to the conclusions she based on these phantasies.

A word about my approach: Hesiod says that the *Theogony* was sung to him by the Muses atop Mt. Helion. I will take this act of creative license as permission to consider and discuss his poem as one might a dream or a phantasy. By this I mean that I accept his vision of the origins, histories, and doings of divine entities not as facts but as a highly elaborated and sometimes imperfectly logical phantasy of aspects of human experience that are not generally accessible to us in our conscious lives. I will approach Klein's suppositions about the unconscious phantasies of infants and young children in a similar spirit. Hesiod thought his phantasy to be of sufficiently universal interest that he made it into a compelling, elaborate, and enduring work of art; Klein made hers into a compelling, elaborate, and – so far – enduring work of psychological theory. The strength of her creative act, like Hesiod's, lies not in logic but in its ability to draw our attention to matters that are generally unnoticed or – more to the point in psychoanalysis – denied.

The *Theogony*: Hesiod's *Theogony* is a mythical genealogy of three generations of gods. More particularly, it is the study of three generations of psychological warfare between divine parents and their divine children, from the expected sibling and triangular rivalries all the way to murder. It is an act of personal creation and the account of an ancient myth – Hesiod's phantasy answer to the universal questions of childhood, a phantasy answer that Klein's clinical experiences make clear, was not his alone. A brief synopsis follows, paraphrased from Richard Caldwell's (1987) translation.

> In the beginning, Hesiod tells us, four divine entities spontaneously emerged into the universe: Chaos, Gaia (or Earth), Tartaros, and Eros. Earth creates for herself a parthenogenetic son and mate whom Hesiod calls Ouranos, or Father-Sky. Together Gaia and Ouranos make many children. But Ouranos fears the rivalrous potential of his children, even while they are still resident in their mother's womb. He therefore keeps them imprisoned within her by mounting her in perpetual intercourse and thereby physically preventing their birth. This becomes too much for Gaia, who cries out in pain and incites the children within her body to plot against their father. Hesiod's gods are immortal and cannot be killed, but Gaia forges a scythe and gives it to her youngest son, Kronos, who castrates Ouranos as he enters her body, thus freeing himself and his siblings.
>
> The second-generation god Kronos, whose name in contemporary Greek means *Time*, although there is contention among scholars as to whether or not Hesiod intended this meaning, chooses for his mate his sister Rhea. Having himself achieved birth by the castration of his father, he has reason to fear the

rivalrous and incestuous desires of his own children. To safeguard his reign, therefore, he swallows them, and so – like his father, although somewhat less sadistically – prevents their emergence as autonomous individuals.

When Kronos's last son is about to be born, Rhea begs her mother's assistance, and she and Gaia trick Kronos by wrapping a stone in a swaddling cloth and giving him this to swallow instead of the newborn. Thus Zeus escapes the fate of his siblings and is hidden by them on a remote island, Crete. Furthermore, the ingestion of the stone causes Kronos to vomit out his other children.

Kronos's rule having been dismantled by his mother and grandmother, a third generation of gods now comes to power. Zeus comes out of his exile in Crete a grown man, but he, like his father and grandfather, fears an unwelcome fate at the hands of his women and children. He therefore swallows whole his pregnant wife Metis, the goddess of intelligence, and by this act of incorporation prevents the birth of rivalrous sons and also acquires her gifts. (When he later gives birth to their daughter Athena, she emerges from his head.) Zeus begets no further legitimate male children, thereby ending the period of the gods' generativity. He installs himself on Mt. Olympos as the final, sole, and omnipotent ruler of the universe.

This summary covers but a small segment of an immensely rich and complex poem. I have had to forgo dozens of the fascinating collateral threads familiar to all of us as the "Greek myths" of our childhoods. Hesiod's vision of the succession story is vastly more complex than Sophocles'. It encompasses not only the familiar terrors of oedipal rivalry but also the terrifying phantasies that Melanie Klein observed in her young child patients: fear of entrapment in the maternal body, dread of parents allied against them, and a vision of perpetual intercourse that debars them from autonomy, inclusion, and perhaps even existence. Klein and Hesiod share a worldview of ruthless parents and conniving children. But whereas he told a story of godly wonders that has enthralled people over millennia, she normalized these tales as the "ordinary" phantasies of mortal childhood.

The convergences matter because they encourage the imaginative expansion of Klein's work, as Sophocles inspired the imaginative expansion of Freud's. Hesiod's storytelling illuminates some still-murky corners of the human character, and any analyst interested enough to read the *Theogony* will find many opportunities to appreciate the insights of this ancient explorer of the rocky shores of relationship.

Parallel Themes in Klein and Hesiod

Prior to Klein, psychoanalysts (with a few exceptions[1]) observed the symptoms, dreams, and associations of their adult patients and intuited from them unconscious childhood phantasies that might have provoked them. Interpreting these "uncovered" phantasies as anxieties, defenses, and conflicts alleviated their patients' symptoms and gave them psychic relief. Melanie Klein treated very young children by interpreting their drawings, their actions, and their play as communications analogous to an adult's free associations. This gave her firsthand access to their phantasies. She engaged the children at their own level, which was often pre-verbal and unsymbolized, and then interpreted to them directly, in a language they could understand, their deepest fears and phantasies, including the negative transference directed toward her as a displacement from primal objects. Interpretation furthered, as it does in work with adults, her child patients' elaboration of the stories that they told their analyst and provided them with great relief as their play unlocked fears, anxieties, hatreds, and envies that could not be addressed otherwise.

Klein insisted on the mother as the first object of desire for children of both genders and located the Oedipus much earlier on the timeline of psychosexual development than in the classical model. She also differed from her Freudian forebears in her embrace of *reparation* rather than dissolution as the means of resolving this complex configuration. Her work expanded the known Freudian repertoire of phantasies, conflicts, and defenses, and established the importance of interpreting the negative transference, and so opened new doors to the understanding of adults and children.

Both Hesiod and Klein offer a wealth of phantasies about where babies come from and how they are born. Here are a few examples of Klein's findings in the context of Hesiod's vision. We see them come together in what I call, in an expansion of Rey's term, the *claustro-agoraphobic dilemma*. This is a group of primitive, infantile phantasies, inferred by Klein and dramatized by Hesiod, of imprisonment in the mother's body or, conversely, forcible exclusion from access to it. Klein believed that all children, normal and psychotic, experience such concerns. Certainly, even a synopsis as brief as mine gives evidence that they were current in ancient Greece millennia before Klein began exploring them in the 1920s. For a comprehensive study of Klein's original notes and drawings of child cases, see Claudia Frank's publication *Melanie Klein in Berlin: Her First Psychoanalyses of Children* (2009).[2]

Endless Parental Intercourse: In the play of Erna, age six, Klein observed an unconscious phantasy of parents engaging in perpetual intercourse. Everything Erna did in the role of her mother, Klein tells us, "had one chief purpose, which was to arouse the child's envy and to wound its feelings" (1932a, p. 39). The imaginary child in Erna's play

> shared its parents' bedroom and had to be a spectator of sexual intercourse between them. If it interrupted it was beaten, and the mother kept on complaining to the father. If she, as the mother, put the child to bed it was only in order to get rid of it and to be able to be united with the father all the sooner. The child was incessantly maltreated and tormented.
>
> (1932a, p. 40)

Combined Parental Couple: Klein presents examples of merged parental phantasies in which penis, nipple, breast, and vagina all combine into one horrifying amalgamation, a frightening vision central in Hesiod as well. Referring to "Early Stages of the Oedipus Complex" (1928), Klein said of her nine-and-a-half-year-old patient,

> Kenneth's fear of his two parents united against him and perpetually copulating with each other proved to be extremely important in his analysis. It was only after I had made many subsequent observations of the same kind in other cases that I realized the fact that fear of "the woman with a penis" is founded upon a sexual theory, formed at a very early stage of development, to the effect that the mother incorporates the father's penis in the act of coitus that I realized the fact that the fear so that as a last resort the woman with a penis signifies the two parents joined together.
>
> (1932b, pp. 102–103)

Children like Erna and Kenneth convinced Klein of a frustrated infant's phantasies that

> father or mother enjoys the desired object of which he is deprived – mother's breast, father's penis – and enjoys it constantly. It is characteristic of the young infant's intense emotions and greed that he should attribute to the parents a constant state of mutual gratification of an oral, anal and genital nature . . . This vision of endless mutual satiation is the foundation for combined parent figures such as: the mother containing the father's penis or the whole father; the father containing the mother's breast or the whole mother; the parents fused inseparably in sexual intercourse.
>
> (1952, p. 79)

Klein made frequent references to her patients' ideas about what can be found within the mother's body: excrement, the father's penis, siblings (often in frightening, monstrous configurations; see, for example, Klein, 1930, p. 219). In particular, she believed that in children's earliest phantasies of parental intercourse, the mother incorporates the father's penis (or his entire body) during the act of coitus. The phantasy of parents so united is a source of massive anxiety in the child, who fears oral sadistic incorporation by them in retaliation for his own sadistic attacks against the mother/breast in nursing (ibid., p. 219).

Castration: Klein's associate Hanna Segal made a telling point relevant to the understanding of all of Klein's cases and also to Hesiod's gods' preoccupation with castration by their children:

> The infant's perception of other people's relationships is very different from the perception of an adult or even an older child. . . . Projections colour all his perceptions. . . . When [an infant] he is under the sway of his own powerful

impulses he phantasies his parents in almost uninterrupted intercourse. . . .
This situation, in which the infant perceives his parents in terms of his own
projections, gives rise to feelings of the most acute deprivation, jealousy, and
envy, since the parents are perceived as constantly giving one another precisely those gratifications which the infant wishes for himself.

(1964a, p. 103)

Klein is referring to such projective attribution when she tells us that sadistic
phantasies about castrating her mother by stealing her babies "were at the bottom
of [Erna's] severe anxiety in regard to her mother. She repeatedly expressed fear
of a 'robber woman' who would 'take out everything inside her'" (1932a, p. 39) –
that is, she feared castration by her mother.

Another example: Rita, almost three years old, played out an obsessional phantasy in which a toy elephant prevented a doll from getting out of bed at night to
harm its parents or to steal from them. She had cast her father as the "preventer,"
Klein says,

ever since, at the time she was a year and a quarter to two years old, she had
wished to usurp her mother's place with him, to steal away the child with
which her mother was pregnant and to injure and castrate both parents.

(1929, p. 202)

Fear of retribution: The violent penetrating phantasies that are such a dramatic
element in Hesiod were found by Klein in both boys and girls. Klein offers as the
reason for them the child's oral envy of the mother's body (and in addition, the
father's penis). "Oral envy is one of the motive forces which make children of
both sexes want to push their way into their mother's body and which arouse the
desire for knowledge allied to it" (1932b, p. 131).

Trude, age three years and nine months, had terrible night terrors and was
incontinent of urine and feces. In play therapy with Klein, Trude had the two of
them pretend that they were both asleep. Then Trude would threaten to stab Klein
in the throat, throw her out the window, burn her, take her to the police. And she
had to look under the rug, which meant, Klein said, "that she wanted to look inside
her mother's bottom for the 'kakis' (faeces), which signified children to her. By
analyzing her wetting and dirtying herself," Klein goes on,

which stood for attacks upon her parents copulating with each other, these
symptoms were removed. Trude had wanted to rob her pregnant mother of
her children, to kill her and to take her place in coitus with her father. She was
two years old when her sister was born.

(1932c, pp. 4–5)

The fear of retribution as represented in the talion law – "an eye for an eye, a
tooth for a tooth" – was as well-known to the early psychoanalysts as it was to

the authors of the Old Testament; Freud, Abraham, Ferenczi, and Jones all recognized it and thought it to represent the unconscious childhood super-ego fears of the adult. In her work with child patients, Klein discovered that such fears arise in *infancy*, that they are operative as unconscious phantasies from birth onward, and that they are particularly harsh in the paranoid-schizoid position of infancy, from birth to 3–4 months. Hesiod too clearly recognized the fear of retribution for deeds and phantasies and depicted it in the Erinyes (the Furies).

Kleinian Development Among the Gods

Let me briefly address a developmental aspect of this material that requires some explanation. Hesiod, mythmaker and dreamer, intuited what the psychoanalyst Klein heard 2,700 years later from her child patients and documented in her reports of their analyses. But he structured his intuition in a literary conceit that may have contributed to its neglect among Klein's colleagues. His parallels with Klein's discoveries about the mental states of young children are more visible and more instructive if we treat his three generations of gods as representing *one* god – that is, one *child* – in development. This child in his infancy is called Ouranos; in early childhood, he appears as Kronos; finally, as he approaches young adulthood, we meet him as Zeus.

In the *Theogony*, Ouranos's paranoid projection of his own murderous wishes results in his castration. Kronos learns enough from his father's story to swallow his own children in an effort to keep himself safe. Zeus, too, absorbs the lessons of the dire father-son battles that preceded his birth. Each generation, with the help of the mother, progresses a little further towards less paranoid and sadistic solutions. Each of these gods assimilates the experiences and learning of the previous generation, as children accomplish their own emotional maturation by absorbing their own pasts.

The Paranoid-Schizoid Position: Ouranos and Kronos exemplify stages of what Klein called the paranoid-schizoid position, a period (from birth to three or four months) during which children cannot distinguish between self and other and are at the mercy of powerful desires and fears. Paranoid and annihilation anxieties dominate as these very young children projectively envision their parents as engaged in perpetual intercourse – that is, constantly satisfying their own desires to the exclusion of their children, and perhaps purposely frustrating, humiliating, and tormenting them.

From three to six months and continuously thereafter, children enter upon the long process of learning to differentiate between self and object, inside and outside, inner reality and external reality. The combined parental couple of the earlier stage can now be conceived of as separate objects, and the matter of whose body parts belong to whom begins to resolve. This new awareness allows for a less persecutory view of the external world than the earlier intellectual and emotional states of the paranoid-schizoid position and also of an internal world – one containing good objects as well as bad – in which children can safely evolve into adulthood. These developments lead children naturally from the paranoid-schizoid position into the depressive position.

The Depressive Position vs. Manic Position: The depressive position brings with it new ego strengths, including a developing capacity for separateness, the capacity to perceive and tolerate ambivalence, and the capacity to bear loss and to mourn. These accomplishments enable the child to see parents as people who can love each other as well as him or her and to tolerate exclusion from the primal couple without the earlier destructive fury. Britton addresses such developments in his essay "The Missing Link," which extends Freud's and Klein's oedipal complex by envisioning the two parents as two sides of the triangle, and the famous third side as the line joining these parents in a mutual relationship (1989). The missing link establishes a triangular space bounded by the three persons of the oedipal situation and all their potential relationships. The capacity to appreciate it represents the closing of the oedipal triangle and the resolution of the complex, and the new perspective informs and enables loving relationships later on.[3] As psychoanalysts generally agree, emotional development requires room, a psychic space, for the other to exist independently of the child's possessive control. This mental consolidation takes place in the depressive position, among whose hallmarks is the appreciation for the parents and their relationship. Also newly acknowledged are the parents' care for the child and gratitude for it, as well as the child's physical and emotional dependence on it. Security in the evolving self and tolerance of being left out grow as the omnipotent child matures into a social being, and sadistic impulses give way in the face of better adaptation and a clearer understanding of psychic and external reality.

These achievements bring new conflicts and other complexities, however, and as the child matures, the twin dangers of enclosure within the maternal body and being shut out of its protection (claustrophobic and agoraphobic anxieties) begin to threaten. The possibility of losing one's mother in retribution for one's own hateful and violent phantasies may be felt as catastrophic anxiety or unbearable guilt. Klein postulates that as they begin to recognize the implications of their reliance on their objects, some children resort to manic defenses (Abraham 1924, pp. 471–474; Klein 1935, 1940) to ward off dependency on the object and to deny the vulnerability to loss. In this state of mind, the child wants to believe that he needs only himself. Unable to tolerate the depressive position's burden of persecutory anxieties and guilt, he forges what Hanna Segal has called defenses of control, triumph, and contempt against the acceptance of his painful situation.

The organization of manic defences in the depressive position includes mechanisms which were already in evidence in the paranoid-schizoid position: splitting, idealization, projective identification, denial, etc. What distinguishes the later use of those defences is that they are highly organized in keeping with the more integrated states of the ego, and that they are specifically directed against the experience of depressive anxiety and guilt.

(1964b, pp. 82–83)

When this occurs, magical thinking and phantasies of omnipotence are enlisted to defeat the unwelcome new awareness of the vulnerable inner and outer worlds. But they leave the manic child alone and lonely; he cannot trust or rely on others to nurture him or allow others to relate to one another or to him. In response to these feelings, he attempts to possess his object (if not inhabit her) through regression to the paranoid-schizoid defense of *projective identification* (Klein 1935, 1940, 1946).

Zeus, the third and last generation of Hesiod's gods, does find his way to the depressive position, but once there, he regresses to Segal's triad of manic defenses as his solution to the problems of dependency and interdependence. His thinking has evolved and matured beyond the sadistic and unrealistic methods of his younger selves (that is, his father and grandfather) in that he seeks prevention rather than dismemberment, imprisonment, or murder. But his solution is as perverse as it is manic. He swallows Metis, his first wife, ensuring his safety by assuming control over the birth of her expected child and by preventing the birth of rivalrous sons. He continues to take on other wives and sires many children, both mortal and immortal, but prevents even the conception of a healthy male heir who might threaten his rule. The swallowing usurps the creative agency and function of women (he gives birth to their daughter Athena himself, through his head), and in that incorporative act of projective identification, he *becomes* the female (and thus a "combined object") himself. But in so doing, Zeus puts an end to the generativity of the gods and so, one might say, to time itself.

This manic outcome lays to rest, up to a point, Zeus's persecutory anxieties. However, he continues to fear his reliance on his mother. While his "rescue" by her – her help in defeating his father – ensures his oedipal triumph, it also raises questions about what she might do to *him*. The countervailing fear of loss, and his guilt in relation to his objects both internal and external, are also felt strongly and manically battled against as he projects his distrust onto all of his "others." Ultimately Zeus ends up challenging the entire universe, filled with the many monster gods his ancestors, including Kronos, Gaia, and Rhea, have created, and he destroys them all. But in so doing, he destroys his remaining family ties. Victorious and without legitimate male offspring, he will rule the universe forever as the last of the gods. He has brought his phallic-manic-omnipotent solution to a triumphant conclusion. But he is alone (Klein 1963).

Claustro-Agoraphobic Fears: Among the wealth of phantasies that Hesiod and Klein offer about where babies come from and how they are born, especially striking are the simultaneous fears of being trapped within the mother's body (claustrophobia) and of being forcibly excluded from it, left unprotected from the dangers without (agoraphobia). Klein thought that this "claustro-agoraphobic syndrome," as Henri Rey later called it (1994, p. 9), occurs in all children, both normal and psychotic. Clearly, such phantasies were current in Greece long before Klein's explorations of the 1920s, and it appears likely that Hesiod's poem includes even earlier aspects of the oral tradition of the Near East, which Hesiod was among the first to compose in the Greek alphabet (Caldwell 1989, pp. 71–74). Furthermore, the need for protection is strongly felt where the organization of triangular rivalries is very flexible as distinctions between the sexes, the generations, and even individuals are not yet reliable, and so castration and invasion phantasies may be aimed at both parents or either one.

The Case of Richard, a Study of Reparation: Klein's case of Richard, age ten, whom she began analyzing during the bombardment of London by the German Luftwaffe in 1939, offers an illuminating picture of the claustro-agoraphobic dilemma and the path out of Hesiodian terrors.

Richard was brought to analysis for being difficult at home and for fearfulness: specifically, school phobia, fear of other children, and fear of going outside. His fears grew worse after a ten-day separation from Klein. When the analysis resumed, Richard's mother reported to Klein a conversation between them: Richard had told his mother that

> he was very worried about having babies later on and had asked her whether it would hurt very much. In reply she had, not for the first time, explained the part played by the man in reproduction, whereupon he had said he would not like to put his genital into somebody else's genital: that would frighten him, and the whole thing was a great worry to him.
>
> (1945, p. 374)

Richard categorized his mother's body (and Klein's) as "a pig-sty with his father's bad penis inside" (ibid., p. 375). This phantasy clarified to Klein some aspects of Richard's anxiety.

> There was a close connection between Richard's fear of his "bad" father's penis inside his mother and his phobia of children. Both these fears were closely bound up with the phantasies about his mother's "inside" as a place of danger. For he felt he had attacked and injured the imaginary babies inside his mother's body, and they had become his enemies. A good deal of anxiety was transferred on to children in the external world.
>
> (Ibid., p. 375)

Klein found evidence in one of Richard's drawings of fears that he was in danger of castration by his father in response to his genital desires towards his mother. Specifically, Richard had drawn a "patrolling" British airplane, suspiciously keeping watch, as Klein saw it, over Richard's desire to oust his father. "I furthermore interpreted that Richard himself had been 'patrolling' his parents, for he was not only inquisitive about their sexual life but unconsciously strongly desired to interfere with it and to separate his parents" (ibid., p. 384).

Unlike Hesiod's gods, however, who had no psychoanalyst to interpret their primitive paranoia and claustro-agoraphobic anxieties, Richard eventually found a way through his fears. Klein's intervention helped him to move into the depressive position of guilt, loss, sorrow, and reparation, where he staggered, as many do, between swaggering attempts at manic repair and genuine emotional reparation. He struggled to relinquish his omnipotent wishes and desires, to make amends for the damage he had done in phantasy to his family members, and to work toward a resolution to, rather than an escape from, the oedipal complex. He had to sacrifice his omnipotence, imperiousness, and other manic denials of reality. But in allowing himself to be a boy rather than a god – to accept the losses of "ordinariness" – he also became able to express wishes to

> restore harmony and peace in the family, by allowing his parents to come together and by giving way to his father's and brother's authority. This implied the need to restrain jealousy and hatred, for only then, he felt, could he avoid the fight with his father for the possession of his mother. In that way he both warded off his castration fear and preserved the good father and the good brother. Above all, he saved his mother from being injured in the fight between father and himself.

> (Ibid., p. 378)

The case of Richard clearly demonstrates Klein's view of how reparation, a depressive-position concept, brings about the conclusion of the oedipal situation and the resolution of claustro-agoraphobic fears. It is also, perhaps, an example of why psychoanalysis matters – for as Zeus shows us, poetry alone is not always enough.

Conclusion

The body of the mother is the foundation of unconscious phantasy in all of us and, therefore, the primary source not only of life but also of our inherent desire for knowledge and its ambiguous payload of pleasure, pain, and frustration. Children's curiosity about what lurks inside the womb/cave (Finkelstein 2016) is a potent force driving them toward mature thinking. In their own ways, Hesiod and Klein both address this curiosity and the terrifying phantasies that even very young children evolve to satisfy it. Both authors pay particular attention to claustrophobic anxieties about entombment within the mother's body (represented variously in Hesiod as Gaia – Earth herself – or the hell-like Tartarus, and in Klein as the mother's womb, anus, or stomach). They also recognize the agoraphobic anxieties of being left unprotected in a dangerous world, expelled from the womb or a nurturing relationship; this is the calamity symbolized by perpetual intercourse between the parents. In children, these two fears are equally terrifying and often coexist.

In 1945 Klein revised her 1928 paper "Early Stages of the Oedipus Complex" to include dependency, guilt, damage done and phantasied, and the need for reparation (that is, the accomplishments of the depressive position), which are the cornerstones of resolution although these concepts were already present in her work with Erna and the other child cases she treated.[4]

This view differed vastly from the Freudian understanding of "dissolution." It is the working through of manic defenses against loss and dependency that enables acceptance of the organizing and integrative aspects of reality, including the parental relationship, as a truth upon which the child's well-being depends.

Hesiod and Klein both portray the fearsome internal landscape of a child struggling to control his own sadistic impulses and the paranoia they beget; Hesiod's poem in particular, we might say, is a work about the horrors of children ensconced in the paranoid-schizoid position. The world they inhabit is menaced, among other things, by an internalized and monstrously combined mother-father, a hideous hybrid that engenders both the terrible fear of being attacked by it and the equally terrifying fear of trying to ward it off by preemptive projective attack.

Both authors honor our curiosity about our own creation, about sex, and about our mothers' bodies. It is worth noting that Klein was the first psychoanalyst to write about children's proto-knowledge of body parts and intercourse; she was also the first to acknowledge openly that children knew more about these things than the adults of her time were willing to give them credit for. Money-Kyrle does make the point that children's cognitive development suffers from "intra-psychic paranoia" and/or "unconscious misconceptions and delusions" about parental intercourse. He writes,

> Where, for example, I would formerly have interpreted a dream as a representation of the parents' intercourse, I would now more often interpret it as a misrepresentation of this event. Indeed, every conceivable representation of it seems to proliferate in the unconscious *except the right one.*
>
> (1968, pp. 416–417)

Nonetheless, Klein's child cases document what we tend to suspect: that children form very early hypotheses about where we come from and how they strive actively to refine and confirm them.

Klein also understood that children perceive these important structures psychologically and physically – the claustrum of the mother, for example, symbolizes both protection and exclusion (Jones 1912, p. 256; Meltzer 2008), while the vagina seeks to take in (that is, introject) the father's external penis, which itself is seeking to enter (that is, project itself into) that opening.

Henri Rey defines psychoanalytic universals as

> the very primitive mechanisms and structures of the mind relevant to psychoanalysis, such as *in utero* processes as well as early baby-mother relationships, to such paranoid-schizoid structures, part-object relationships, depressive processes and also the early elaboration of inner space, consisting of inner and external objects.
>
> (1994, p. 1)

They include anxieties about life and death, phantasies about physical bodies and processes, and relationships. They are the recurrent beliefs and fears of small children – the ones found in psychoanalysis and in fairy tales – and in myths.

Klein and Hesiod, from their different points of view, articulate the universal phantasies of curious children about life *in utero* and the sexual actualities that bring it about. The mother's body is the primary focus of the infant's life, and preoccupations about its inner and outer reality are the primary focus of early phantasy. Until the child becomes able to differentiate himself from his objects and psychic reality from the "real" world, "inside" spaces and "outside" spaces remain indistinguishable, and claustro-agoraphobic and other paranoid fears cannot be escaped.

The claustrophobic fear of being imprisoned within the mother and the agoraphobic wish to return to the womb and fear of being shut out of it are themes of which dreams and nightmares are made, and Hesiod's great work is proof positive that they are more than psychoanalytic chimeras. They really *are* universal longings and conflicts that have contributed to the mental development of humankind for thousands of years.

Notes

1 Hermine von Hug-Hellmuth (whose "play technique" Klein borrowed and modified) was one of these exceptions, as of course was Anna Freud. However, neither Hug-Hellmuth nor Anna Freud interpreted directly to children the meaning of the negative transference or their unconscious phantasies.
2 For a comprehensive study of Klein's child cases in the 1920s with original case notes and drawings, see Claudia Frank's *Melanie Klein in Berlin Her First Psychoanalyses of Children* (2009), Routledge: London.
3 As with all developmental gains, of course, these are not absolute. Adults as well as children may alternate between these two positions in times of stress. Once the classical Oedipus complex is reached and worked through, however, newly achieved ego strength leaves the individual better able to negotiate the formerly crippling anxieties of the paranoid-schizoid position.
4 See Klein and Riviere (1936) *Love, Hate and Reparation*, by Klein and Joan Riviere, for a comprehensive understanding of early primitive unconscious processes of love, hate, and reparation in infancy and adulthood already known in the child cases from the 1920s and 1930s.

References

Abraham, K. (1924). A Short Study of the Development of the Libido Viewed in the Light of Mental Disorders. In *Selected Papers of Karl Abraham, M.D.* (1949, D. Bryan and A. Strachey, Trans.). Hogarth.

Britton, R. (1989). The Missing Link: Parental Sexuality in the Oedipus Complex. In R. Britton, M. Feldman, and E. O'Shaughnessy (Eds), *The Oedipus Complex Today*. Karnac.

Britton, R. (1992). The Oedipus Situation and the Depressive Position. In R. Anderson (Ed.), *Clinical Lectures on Klein and Bion*. Routledge, pp. 34–45.

Caldwell, R. (1987). *Hesiod's Theogony*. Focus Classical Library.

Caldwell, R. (1989). *The Origin of the Gods*. Oxford University Press.

Finkelstein, S. (2016). Psychosomatic Illness in a Claustro-Agoraphobic Patient. In P.L. Sloate (Ed.), *From Soma to Symbol*. Karnac.

Jones, E. (1912). A Forgotten Dream: Note on the Oedipus Saving Phantasy (1923 Edition). In *Papers on Psycho-Analysis* (3rd Edition, pp. 255–265). Baillere, Tindall and Cox.

Klein, M. (1928). Early Stages of the Oedipus Conflict (1975 Edition). In *Love, Guilt, and Reparation and Other Works: 1921–1945*. Free Press.

Klein, M. (1929). Personification in the Play of Children (1975 Edition). In *Love, Guilt, and Reparation and Other Works, 1921–1945*. Free Press.

Klein, M. (1930). The Importance of Symbol-Formation in the Development of the Ego (1975 Edition). In *Love Guilt and Reparation and Other Works, 1921–1945*. Free Press.

Klein, M. (1932a). An Obsessional Neurosis in a Six-Year-Old Girl (1975 Edition). In *The Psychoanalysis of Children, Part I: The Technique of Child Analysis* (A. Strachey, Trans.). Hogarth.

Klein, M. (1932b). The Effects of Early Anxiety-Situations on the Sexual Development of the Boy (1975 Edition). In *The Psychoanalysis of Children, Part I: The Technique of Child Analysis* (A. Strachey, Trans.). Hogarth.

Klein, M. (1932c). The Technique of Analysis in the Latency Period (1975 Edition). In *The Psychoanalysis of Children, Part I: The Technique of Child Analysis* (A. Strachey, Trans.). Hogarth.

Klein, M. (1935). A Contribution to the Psychogenesis of Manic-Depressive States (1975 Edition). In *Love, Guilt, and Reparation and Other Works: 1921–1945*. Free Press.

Klein, M. (1940). Mourning and Its Relation to Manic-Depressive States (1975 Edition). In *Love, Guilt, and Reparation and Other Works: 1921–1945*. Free Press.

Klein, M. (1945). The Oedipus Complex in the Light of Early Anxieties (1975 Edition). In *Love, Guilt, and Reparation and Other Works: 1921–1945*. Free Press.

Klein, M. (1946). Notes of Some Schizoid Mechanisms (1975 Edition). In M. Masud and R. Khan (Ed.), *Envy and Gratitude and Other Works: 1946–1963*. Free Press.

Klein, M. (1952). Some Theoretical Conclusions Regrading the Emotional Life of the Infant (1975 Edition). In M. Masud and R. Khan (Ed.), *Envy and Gratitude and Other Works: 1946–1963*. Free Press.

Klein, M. (1963a). On the Sense of Loneliness (1975 Edition). *Envy and Gratitude and Other Works: 1946–1963*. Free Press, pp. 300–313.

Klein, M. (1963b). Some Reflections on *The Oresteai*. *Envy and Gratitude and Other Works: 1946–1963* (1975 Edition). Free Press, pp. 275–299.

Klein, M., and Riviere, J. (1936). *Love, Hate and Reparation*. W.W. Norton & Company.

Meltzer, D. (2008). *The Claustrum*. Karnac.

Money-Kyrle, R.E. (1968). Cognitive Development. *International Journal of Psychoanalysis. 49*, 691–698.

Rey, H. (1994). The Schizoid Mode of Being and the Space-Time Continuum (Before Metaphor). In J. Magnana (Ed.), *Universals of Psychoanalysis in the Treatment of Psychotic and Borderline States*. Free Association Books.

Segal, H. (1964a). The Early Stages of the Oedipus Complex. In *Introduction to the Work of Melanie Klein*. Basic Books.

Segal, H. (1964b). Manic Defenses. In *Introduction to the Work of Melanie Klein*. Basic Books.

Chapter 10

Claustro-Agoraphobia

The Impact of Concrete Thinking on the Analyst's Internal Space[1]

Heinz Weiss

SUMMARY

Heinz Weiss examines the claustro-agoraphobic dilemma in the context of his work on borderline patients and pathological organizations of the personality (Weiss 2009). The concepts of time and space play an important role in his thinking. He often refers to John Steiner's (1993) theory of 'psychic retreats', which he describes as timeless states of mind. In his recent book *Trauma, Guilt and Reparation* (Weiss 2020), Weiss describes pathological organizations figuring as 'dungeons', 'towers', or 'desolate islands'. They initially serve as safe havens, which protect the patient from unbearable fear and pain, but later on transform into prisons, which are difficult to escape. In his contribution, he refers to the ideas of Bion (1962), Segal (1957), Steiner (1993), and Rey (1979). Presenting detailed clinical material, he emphasizes the role of concrete thinking in claustro-agoraphobia and its impact on the analyst's internal space. He explores the role of the analyst's counter-transference and argues that a transition from concrete to symbolic thinking is only possible when reparative processes emerge.

TEXT

Introduction

As shown in the previous chapters of this book, claustro-agoraphobia delineates an area where the individual can tolerate neither intimacy nor separateness without feeling trapped, confused, or abandoned. Claustro-agoraphobic problems are regarded as resulting from a specific difficulty of the individual – often due to early traumatic experiences (Weiss 2020) or lack of containment – to construct his or her mental space. It has far-reaching consequences on the individual's interpersonal relationships, sense of identity, capacity for symbolic thinking, and experience of time. It also affects the experience of the body because emotional experiences, which cannot be processed and symbolized, often persist as bizarre bodily sensations or hypochondriac anxieties.

DOI: 10.4324/9781003200284-10

Another phenomenon, which is quite common in patients with claustro-agoraphobic anxieties, is the persistence of a cruel, archaic super-ego and the difficulty to make reparation or develop a capacity for forgiveness. The connection between concrete thinking, disturbances of the space-time continuum, and the dominance of a cruel super-ego is an area that still needs further exploration.

Amongst the authors who have described different aspects of claustro-agoraphobia Donald Meltzer's (1966, 1992) work on the 'claustrum' and 'geographical confusion' and Henri Rey's (1979) exploration of the 'claustro-agoraphobic dilemma' (1979) are of particular significance.[2] With the latter term, Rey depicts the impasse the individual feels exposed to when they are able to tolerate neither closeness nor distance, as well as the permanent thread to their sense of identity through anxieties of a paranoid-schizoid or depressive kind. According to Rey (1979, 1994a, 1994b), claustro-agoraphobic anxieties are prominent in schizoid and borderline individuals but also occur in neurotic and psychotic patients (Steiner 1993; Weiss 2009). The situation in which the individual feels trapped often ends up in despair. It gives rise to repetitive cycles because the subject feels that she or he has 'nowhere a place'.

In his work, Rey has put special emphasis on the role of concrete thinking and the availability of a 'marsupial space' to transform concrete objects into symbolic meaning and to develop the individual's internal space. In my contribution, I want to explore these aspects, namely the *concreteness of the claustro-agoraphobic patient's communications* due to a lack of symbol formation (Segal 1957, 1978) and *the pressure they exert on others by intruding into their mental space*. I will argue that this has the temporary effect of *numbing* our thinking (Bion 1952; Steiner 2014 [2011]) and deforming the analyst's mental space before we can regain a capacity for symbolic thinking. If we succeed in doing so, we may provide our internal space, as Rey says, as a 'marsupial space' for the patient.

Clinical Material

Mr T, a 40-year-old IT assistant, came to see me when he was in a depressed mood, fearing he could become mad. He had been in analytic treatment already several times. However, all these treatments had ended in a deadlock and finally been broken off because, as he said, the therapists could no longer 'stand' him. Therefore, he was not sure whether I could 'stand' him, and for that reason, he withheld information on parts of his history – in particular, a longer psychotic breakdown when he was at university in his early 20s. He was afraid that, like his previous therapists, I would find him 'intolerable', and if I terminated his analysis, he said, nobody would accept him anymore, and he would be exposed to loneliness, madness, or death.

History

Mr T had been brought up in a family with parents who were extreme opposites but lived together in a kind of forced marriage. Both belonged to the same religious sect. The rules and demands of the sect dominated the atmosphere in the family. Mr T said that the children were forced to work like slaves on the parent's farm. They had to pray before breakfast, and any transgression of the family rules was punished in a ritualized way.

There was some indication that Mr T's mother, who came from an urban background, was chronically unhappy and depressed. He described her gaze as cold and rejecting and supposed that she accused her children of her destiny to have to live with the father and his parents on the farm. He remembered that during his childhood, she would sometimes run away and that there was a fear that she would never return or even kill herself. The father was described as a warmer person but, in his reactions, often choleric towards the mother and the children.

Mr T was the second of five children. His childhood reminiscences were somehow incoherent and dispersed, shifting between spells of romantic idealization and an overall atmosphere of duty, discipline, and fear. He described his parents as permanently quarrelling with each other, and he conveyed an impression that no one realized how timorous, isolated, and depressed he grew up. In order to overcome his family background, he tried to excel at school and was successful in getting access to a renowned university.

There was a narrative that he was cyanotic after birth due to an umbilical cord enlacement and that his mother was terrified to see him like this. This, together with his panic/fear that she could run away and never return, seemed to stand for his claustro-agoraphobic fear of being either strangled or abandoned. There was also a reminiscence that it was difficult to feed him and that he was underweight during his childhood.

In Mr T's adolescence, his older sister died in a car accident. This triggered the first period of confusion. At university, he joined a religious students' fraternity from which he was finally expelled because of his mistrust, withdrawal, and provocative behaviour. Subsequently, he suffered a psychotic breakdown, which required psychiatric inpatient treatment for several months. Eventually, he succeeded in finishing his degree and found work in the IT department of a large firm.

In his adult life, Mr T had never been able to hold down a job or an intimate personal relationship for a longer time. There were often doubts about the inadequacy of his body and his 'masculinity'. He had never had a partner, often felt misunderstood, was treated unfairly, and in consequence, reacted reproachfully or by withdrawing into a cold distance. Emotional intimacy went along with mistrust and fear, while experiences of loss often ended up in confusion or despair. He could neither be alone nor share a space with another person. Frequently he was caught up in power struggles in which he felt hurt and maltreated, not realizing to what degree he could himself behave arrogantly and dismissive towards others. In a similar way, he could not stand to stay alone in his flat but would complain about having 'no home' when travelling around.

Behaviour During Therapy

As might be expected, we soon experienced similar difficulties in the analytic encounter. Mr T did not know how to begin the session or would sort out what he did not want to let me know. Then he would speak in minute detail about the arguments he had had with a colleague and his difficulties in furnishing his flat, and he would complain about the tax authorities, the doctors who treated him badly, and the confrontations with his garage or his insurance. During these lengthy statements, I was not allowed to intervene, and when I did try to say something after 20 or 30 minutes, he would angrily remark that I should stop interrupting him. If I did manage to make a comment, he did not pick up on it but just continued speaking where he left off. At the end of the session, he would complain that, yet again, he had not been able to address what he had wanted to speak about.

Such behaviour made me feel helpless and angry. If he felt my anger, he complained that I forced my ideas on him, wronging and humiliating him. He announced he would make an official complaint about me. My narcissism, he said, would be well known; the sparrows would 'whistle it from the roofs'. In this occasion, I felt so provoked that I replied he saw himself as the sparrow high up on the roof, looking down on me. But such retaliation only led to further escalations. Then his mood would collapse, and he would fall into despair, fearing that I would see him as a 'hopeless case' and terminate his treatment. At the same time, he hinted that he could not survive without the sessions. Yet on no account was I allowed to understand this as an indication of his neediness or dependency.

Between sessions or during holiday breaks, he sent me long emails but did not expect me to reply to them. In doing so, his main intention seemed to be to get rid of something that he wanted to deposit inside me. He said that he did not allow himself to think about my person because he feared these thoughts would remain in him without being able to expel them. He might then lose control, and that would make him even more desperate and lonesome.

There was a similar problem when I addressed his relationship with me in the session. He saw transference interpretations as 'provocations' in which I invaded him, expelling him from a protected space that belonged exclusively to him. Then he complained that he was unable to think. He became confused and demanded in a harsh tone of voice that I should 'definitely stop that'. When the tension became unbearable, he would stand up and leave the consulting room in utter indignation, only to return a few minutes later asking whether he could continue. He seemed to fear that I would take revenge and not allow him to return or throw him out. Such behaviour sometimes repeated itself several times within a session. He often postponed important issues right up to the end of the session and then feared there was no time left to communicate them. There were similar problems at the beginning of the session when he worried that he had mixed up the time of the session, not locked the door of his flat, or even taken the wrong bus so that he arrived in a rush and just in time. In all this, he meticulously observed my reactions and noted my state of mind very precisely, even before I was aware of it myself.

For a long time, Mr T's analysis was characterized by a lack of dreams. Even the thoughts he had wanted to talk about sometimes 'disappeared' when he had entered the room. In the second year, he let me know about a pictorial phantasy which had tormented him for many years. In this phantasy, he saw a rat imprisoned in a crib. The animal was threatened by knives stabbing at her through slits in the crib. So the rat had no choice but to snap and bite back.

This was, of course, a terrible picture, but it seemed to illustrate quite accurately the transference situation as Mr T perceived it.

In the third year, he mentioned fragments of dreams but was unable to recollect them. Eventually, he mentioned a dream in which 'things' were put into a microwave, making it explode.

I suggested that he saw his thoughts as dangerous 'things' that he wanted to deposit inside me but feared that I would 'burst'. Nevertheless, by telling me this dream, he had found a way to communicate his fears and overcome the blockage in his thinking.

In another dream, he was offered a cake that was made out of pieces of older cakes and other indigestible material.

When I suggested that he saw my interpretations as forcing something indigestible back into him, he promptly confirmed, 'Exactly, you form certain "pieces" from what I said, mix it up with other material and bits of theory into something I can't eat and that makes me vomit.' Thus, he seemed to feel that I made him eat his own vomit, which reminded me of the feeding problems in his childhood.

This was a particularly difficult period in his analysis where we would often get into confrontations. Sometimes I felt that I got angry, insisted on what I had said, and then was actually forcing something back into him. Often, we found ourselves in a deadlock, and any attempt to explore his part in the escalating conflicts was experienced as a mistake or attack on my part. Mistakes were dangerous and could lead to explosions or punishment. Thus, we found ourselves in a world where there was little space for thinking, reparation, or understanding. The overall atmosphere seemed dominated by a cruel super-ego, which insisted on punishment and guilt, and I tried to imagine how he might have experienced the religious indoctrination by his parents. I also thought about the possible link between his running away from the sessions and his mother's running away from the parents' home.

Material From a Session

Despite all these difficulties, there was some progress in the fourth and fifth years of Mr T's analysis. His professional situation had improved. He had changed his post, and he described his new chief as a more appreciative and friendly figure. With his support, he had become a team manager, which confronted him with new responsibilities. For the first time, he had met a girlfriend with whom he spent a week of holidays, though he was still not able to share a room with her. At that time, his father had to undergo surgery, and he visited his parents every weekend.

This coincided with the Easter break, and sometimes, he seemed to be sad and missed our sessions.

He continued to have difficulties furnishing his apartment. After careful consideration, he had finally opted for a sofa that had now to be delivered and set up. As the date of delivery coincided with his working time and our session, he had left the keys with his neighbour and asked the furnisher company to set up the sofa in his flat.

He arrived at his session in a rush and 20 minutes late. He explained that he had been stuck in a traffic jam but had also been on the phone with the furniture company. He felt distressed: it might all go wrong. He went on to describe the complicated situation in detail and then complained about missing out on the part of the session.

After this, he mentioned a dream from the night before in which his landlord had explained to him that his flat had been moved to a bigger building. It was an apartment in a modern multi-storey house, furnished in a functional, slightly cold, but aesthetic style. Inside the apartment, there was a couch with a stove in the background which warmed up the room.

When he said this, I had some thoughts about the building, the couch, and the warmer atmosphere.

He added that I would probably expect associations from him, but he had none. Last night, he woke up and wept because he felt so lonely. But now he had to concentrate on his work and the delivery of his sofa. This must not go wrong and was of utmost importance.

At that moment, I felt like one of the delivery men he had phoned on his way to the session, and when I just wanted to make a comment, his mobile phone rang.

He apologized but instantly explained he *had to receive* this call because it was so important.

Thus I became witness to a ten-minute phone conversation which he conducted from the couch. I learned that something had gone wrong. The delivery men stood in front of his locked door. The neighbour to whom he had committed the key was not there. He became desperate and did not know what to do.

He felt embarrassed that he had received the call and had phoned for so long. But the problem of how to move the sofa in, he explained, had absolute priority. It seemed to him almost irresolvable because the door was locked. He regretted having lost another part of the session, and now the situation between the two of us seemed similarly intractable like the problem in his flat.

I felt excluded during his phone call but decided to understand the scene as a continuation of his dream or as an association with it. Therefore, I said he wanted me to help him to move something into him but felt terribly afraid it could go wrong.

For a moment, he listened attentively to what I was saying. But then he explained that the most important thing was to find a solution to the problem with his sofa. His idea was that the delivery men could assemble it in the hallway outside his flat, and when his neighbour arrived, he could move it into his flat. But would that work? Was the door wide enough for the sofa to fit through? And how could it be that the neighbour wasn't there? Hadn't he trusted him with the key?

I suggested that he would find himself in an awkward position if he trusted me to help him – the neighbour's help to whom he had confided the key – but I could not go on with what I was saying because he became more and more despairing and interrupted me.

He said that if the sofa was assembled *outside* his flat and moved in afterwards, it would be no longer *his* sofa.

I replied that he feared that if he deposited his thoughts inside me, they would be no longer *his* but rather force them as *my thoughts* back into him. At the same time, I felt I could no longer reach him, that he was 'locked', and I no longer had access to his internal space – just like the delivery men who were standing outside in front of a locked door.

Thus, the session ended with regret and utter confusion.

Discussion

Reflecting on this session, I thought that it illustrates the difficulty of moving from a form of communication, which is equated with the transposition of 'facts' to an understanding of their meaning. Both Mr T and I felt under pressure, although it was not the *same* pressure, and we were pursuing *different objectives.*

His main objective was that the delivery of his sofa should not go wrong. For that reason, he had phoned the furnishing company on the way to the session, which had contributed to his delay. He seemed preoccupied with the time of delivery and the assembly of his sofa. Then he told me about his dream in which his apartment had been displaced to a modern, functional building. There was a couch with a stove in the background, which conveyed a sense of warmth and cosiness.

This contrasted with the hectic, agitated mood in which he had arrived. He claimed that he had no associations with his dream but then mentioned his sadness when he woke up realizing how lonely he felt.

I saw this in connection to the Easter break that had just taken place and to his fear that his father might die. The multi-storey building corresponded to the building where his analysis took place, and of course, the sofa in the dream evoked the thought of the couch in the consulting room.

All this conveyed an idea about the *symbolic meaning* of his communication. However, before I could make a comment, he stepped back to the level of 'facts', letting me know that the most important thing right now was the delivery of his sofa.

Thus, in a very concrete way, the *exchange of ideas* was substituted with *facts* and experienced by Mr T as the moving of furniture into a locked room.

This impression was confirmed when he conducted a long phone call with the delivery men, which made me feel excluded from his internal space. I tried to overcome this feeling by seeing the phone call as a continuation of his dream, so to say, as an association to it, as if he wanted to make me feel how *he* experienced our relationship.

For a moment, he listened to my interpretation attentively but quickly returned to the domain of 'facts' where the most urgent problem was whether the sofa could be set up outside the flat. Would the door be wide enough to pass it through? And had confiding the key to the neighbour been a trap?

I think he was dealing with feelings of being excluded during the Easter break and with sadness and fears about losing his father. Probably he was also struggling with the fears that were emerging when a warmer atmosphere had developed between us in the sessions, and he had begun to trust me. Could he find a safe place inside me after returning, or would he be trapped? Would his thoughts then still belong to him, or would I instead put my thoughts into him just like a piece of furniture?

At the end of the session, we seemed to speak about the *same issue* but not in the *same language*. However, both his regret and also my feelings of helplessness certainly differed from the rat's struggle for survival in the crib. I also think he no longer considered my thoughts to be 'poisoned food' but expressed some of his own sadness and helplessness by evoking these feelings in me.

In the next session, I learned that the problem with the sofa had been resolved. He recalled his parents' attempts to 'convert' him to their belief system, how he had turned away from them in his youth, how lonely he had felt at university, and that there had once been an elusive feeling that perhaps, one day, things would turn out well. At this moment, it seemed clear that he did not see me pushing my interpretations like dogma into him but wished to internalize something warm and soft and someone to keep the door open for him.[3] However, in the following session, new problems emerged: he had been cut off from electricity because he hadn't checked his post and overlooked the invoice and reminders that had been sent to him.

Conclusion

In this paper, I have tried to depict some of the difficulties which result from the analyst being drawn into the patient's claustro-agoraphobic dilemma. This can take the form of re-enactments or of a 'numbing' of the analyst's thinking. In any case, he must deal with the problem that the patient is putting raw, non-symbolized elements into him, which he has to contain, gradually transform, and finally return in a less indigestible form to the patient (see Bion 1962; Steiner 2014 [2011]).

When the analyst's mind is filled up with all this raw material, his internal space becomes temporarily deformed. With the onset of reparative mechanisms on the part of the analyst, it may be restored and, at best, be transformed into a marsupial space (Rey 1979) for the patient. I think that this *temporary deformation* frequently occurs in patients with serious claustro-agoraphobic problems. Theoretically, it can be conceptualized as resulting from the projection of highly condensed, non-symbolized part-object relations. The intensity of these projections creates tensions which affect our capacity for thinking. Perhaps one could picture them as intra-psychic 'gravitation waves' to gain a better understanding of the explosive pressure and the implosive pull to which patient and analyst feel exposed in the transference and counter-transference.

Notes

1 Parts of the clinical material are also published in the International Journal of Psycho-Analysis, vol. 103, no. 3 (2022), doi.org/10.1080/00207578.2022.2060482 (online publication).
2 See Chapters 5 and 7 in this book.
3 I wish to thank John Steiner (London) for this comment.

References

Bion, W.R. (1952). Group Dynamics: A Re-view. In: Bion, W.R. (Ed.), *Experiences in Groups and Other Papers* (1959, 1961 Edition). Heinemann.

Bion, W.R. (1962). *Learning from Experience* (1990 Edition). Heinemann.

Meltzer, D. (1966). The Relation of Anal Masturbation to Projective Identification. *International Journal of Psychoanalysis. 47,* 335–342.

Meltzer, D. (1992). *The Claustrum. An Investigation of Claustrophobic Phenomena.* Clunie Press.

Rey, H. (1994a). *Universals of Psychoanalysis in the Treatment of Psychotic and Borderline States* (J. Magagna, Ed.). Free Association.

Rey, H. (1994b). Basic Schizoid Structures and Space-time Factors. In: Rey, H., and Magagna, J. (Eds), *Universals of Psychoanalysis in the Treatment of Psychotic and Borderline States.* (pp. 163–175). Free Association.

Rey, J.H. (1979). Schizoid Phenomena in the Borderline Syndrome. The Schizoid Mode of Being and the Space-time Continuum. In: Rey, H., (1994) and Magagna, J. (Eds), *Universals of Psychoanalysis in the Treatment of Psychotic and Borderline States* (pp. 8–30). Free Association.

Segal, H. (1957). Notes on Symbol Formation. *International Journal of Psychoanalysis. 38,* 391–397.

Segal, H. (1978). On Symbolism. *International Journal of Psychoanalysis. 59,* 315–319.

Steiner, J. (1993). *Psychic Retreats: Pathological Organizations in Psychotic, Neurotic and Borderline Patients.* Routledge.

Steiner, J. (2014 [2011]). Das betäubende Gefühl von Wirklichkeit. In: Steiner, J., Weiß, H., and Frank, C. (Eds), *Seelische Rückzugsorte verlassen: Therapeutische Schritte zur Aufgabe der Borderline-Position* (pp. 77–96). Klett-Cotta.

Weiss, H. (2009). *Das Labyrinth der Borderline-Kommunikation: Klinische Zugänge zum Erleben von Raum und Zeit.* Klett-Cotta.

Weiss, H. (2020). *Trauma, Guilt and Reparation: The Path from Impasse to Development.* Routledge.

Chapter 11

Intimacy and Loss of Orientation[1]

Claudia Frank

SUMMARY

In her contribution, Claudia Frank explores Roger Money-Kyrle's (1968) concept of 'disorientation' both as a means to get lost and trapped inside an object through projective identification and an attempt to escape from frightening intimacy. Money-Kyrle has coined the term 'misconceptions of reality', which he connects with the three 'basic facts of life': the acknowledgement of the dependency on the breast as an external source of goodness; the recognition of parental intercourse as a creative act, which generates new life; and the acceptance of transience and ultimately death (Money-Kyrle 1971). Frank gives a detailed clinical account of her patient who was caught in a vicious cycle between avoiding meaningful contact (the 'cutter') and his terror of ending and loss. She shows that the 'solution' the patient had found was a perverse one (the 'stirrer', who played with fire) and how his dilemma resonated with the transference and counter-transference. Frank's clinical approach shows traces of the thinking of Edna O'Shaughnessy, who developed her ideas in the midst of Melanie Klein's and Roger Money-Kyrle's work. In particular, her exploration of defensive organisations, of 'enclaves' and 'excursions', where the patient takes refuge, is a poignant description of claustro-agoraphobic situations (O'Shaughnessy 1981, 1992). Claudia Frank is famous for her pioneering work on Klein's first child analysis (1999), where she became familiar with primitive phantasies of a claustro-agoraphobic kind.

TEXT

In patients with a massive claustro-agoraphobic dilemma, who can neither tolerate closeness nor separateness, disorientation can be chosen as an escape from frightening intimacy, which they so much long for at the same time. Taking the example of the analysis of Mr A, I shall explore the explosive area of intimacy in such a patient. As soon as my patient felt a moment of direct encouraging contact on the phone, he felt driven to do anything but come and thus arrived 25 minutes late to his first interview. Discussing material from the analysis of that patient, in

DOI: 10.4324/9781003200284-11

the panic of a burnout syndrome, caught up in a vicious circle of feeling driven to avoid in a hectic way any meaningful contact and work and then being in terror of the end of work, marriage, and indeed life, I will show the precarious work to recognize and differentiate the mental states, connected with the nature of the object experienced. Roger Money-Kyrle's fundamental concepts of orientation and disorientation are helpful in conceptualizing the issues in transference and counter-transference. We see how pathological projective identifications keep up the pathological organization, with excitement by perverse elements when triumphing over an option of some more work in the analytic situation, followed by persecution of losing any basis.

Starting With a Claustro-agoraphobic Enactment

My friendly voice on the phone more than a year ago when Mr A first made contact with me had encouraged him to try me again, he explained when he approached me a second time. Then, I told him that I had no vacancies at present but might be able to offer him a space if he wanted to contact me later on. Now I offered a first appointment, for which he arrived about 25 minutes late, explaining that he was terribly sorry, but he had not thought that there would be so many traffic jams. He could speak about how 'queasy' he felt (as if he was 'going to be cornered'), but these words hardly described his anxious tension. When I described that he looked for help but seemed to be quite fearful of actually meeting me, he would not admit it directly, but it became clear during the initial consultations that he had enacted his problem straightforward with claustrophobia causing his missing the first half and thus robbing us of a shared fuller experience and being simultaneously in a panic to lose a chance for coming to terms with what persecuted him. Several previous attempts of getting help had already petered out.

Mr A was a smart manager, intelligent, and gifted – always trying to negate his anxious state (which I could see and sense). He had changed jobs to 'solve' issues but, in his late 30s, could no longer deny that it was something in him and not primarily in the external world, which seemed 'toxic'. He felt he was heading for a breakdown. He could not but answer every request from his boss with 'No problem!' even though he could envisage the possible problems arising from the realization of the projects. He attempted to calm himself by saying 'somehow' things would work out. But actually, the consequence was that he was 'rotating' 24/7. Despite his hectic endeavours, he was frequently unable to meet deadlines, or the results were unsatisfactory as the requests had been unrealistic in the first place. He knew that if he were able to set out the problems at the start, it would be highly likely that a realistic, mutually agreed plan was possible. But he could just not manage to do this.

There were similar issues at home. For example, he promised to be home early in the evening, although he knew this to be impossible given his timetable. Usually, as the day went on, he reversed his decision bit by bit, saying he might be a bit later than expected, but he was sure he would be back by a certain time.

Eventually, it became clear to him that he would have to stay overnight on his way home, or he would only return the next evening. Now his wife was no longer prepared to tolerate this kind of behaviour. One of his sisters-in-law had benefitted from an analysis, and this is how the idea arose that he might be able to do something for himself in a similar fashion. That made sense to him, but he had not been able to realize it so far. And it became clear during the fourth assessment consultation how he handled the agoraphobic dilemma facing analysis: while he described himself as 'addicted to harmoniousness', he realized, as he said, that he had 'completely forgotten' to bring the application form for the health insurance company, which he had applied for.

The background remained vague in many respects: his much elder brothers had recently found out, he said, that his mother had suffered from depression, and there were a few memories from childhood which might 'fit'. In his late teens, his mother had suffered from locked-in syndrome, was looked after by his father until she died, but was avoided in terror by him. And thereafter also, contact with his father had petered out. That gave an idea of how the claustro-agoraphobic dilemma, described by Henri Rey (1979), came about: either trapped in a deathly container with no proper function of helping psychic growth by symbolizing or being exposed in a shattered world, with no nurture for development, but instead having to keep persecution at bay. Would it be possible for him to allow enough contact for us to work together when his way had been so much one of continuing to expect that his deep-rooted ambivalence would 'somehow' be resolved?

He was stuck in a claustro-agoraphobic dilemma for quite some time while relying – unacknowledged – on objects who cared. The latter seemed to feel increasingly exploited by his more and more excessive use of it. There was – as I heard and felt it – a search to find rest in a 'true' intimate situation and an urgent need to understand what hindered it. And at the same time, I was not quite sure whether it was really his need (or more that of his wife). For me, the fact that he had contacted me a second time indicated something in him that was actively seeking to orient himself towards a friendlier world. It became clear that this was a thin thread when he subsequently missed half of the first assessment interview. But at least the thread was not broken and had not disappeared, even though something disquietingly anti- or un-social was present. The addiction to 'harmoniousness' seemed to be more of an 'addiction' to be in accord with 'not having to' rather than with a close, alive togetherness. At the same time, he was shocked by his mistake of the 'total forgetting' and was absolutely punctual for his next appointment, bringing all the required health insurance documents. In this way, we reached an arrangement for analysis four times a week, on the understanding that he might, on occasion, be unable to make use of all the sessions due to business reasons.

Thus, in contrast to his earlier attempts to get help, we arrived at an agreement due to, I think, my addressing the contradictory movements from the start, trying to hold him with 'two hands' (Brenman Pick 1995), meaning addressing both the patient's vulnerability and his hindering and destructive impulses.

Realizing Disorientation – to Re-Train 'the Cutter in Order to Have Him on the Right Side'

The world of work dominated the sessions in the first few months with his fast, hectic flow of speech describing, on the one hand, his good intentions and, on the other, complaints about his boss fed by indignation and resentment. He seemed driven in every way with few possibilities to establish meaningful contact. One of the rare, more immediate moments happened after the first holiday break. He told me in the first session thereafter that he suffered from a 'stumbling heart'. He tried hard to play down the fear of death he had experienced but had conveyed that the physical investigation, where no pathology had been found, had not really calmed him. When I made a link with my leaving/abandoning him that this might have made his heart stumble, he said he had 'not thought of it like that'. But his heart began to beat regularly again.

Thus, there seemed – on a vegetative level – an essential hold by our setting, with immediate consequences when it was interrupted. My continuous describing his 'good intentions' here in coming to his sessions on the one hand, and then feeling driven to run into all those words in order not to feel what it is like to be here which gave rise to so many complaints, seemed to maintain a basic reassurance, on which he depended. 'Under cover', so to speak, he could allow some work to be done. Breaks interrupted that and so felt to be life-threatening. Linking his symptom with my absence seemed to reach him and thus restore 'his heart'. He fell ill during the next break, too, ending in having to have a surgical intervention of a huge abscess on his back. We could reconstruct that he had behaved as somebody not caring about icy weather – identified with his analyst, whom he unconsciously felt did not care when leaving. But it was hard to grasp something of it more directly as soon as we were again in our 'normal' setting, with his driven state dominating, seldom allowing to be addressed 'effectively'.

Mr A had been in analysis for eight months when, towards the end of a Friday session, the patient stumbled on what he had said. Once again, he talked about preferring to stay in a hotel overnight after he finished his work because 'there were no more musts'. He did not have to talk to his wife or put his little boy to bed. He did not do anything for himself in the hotel, as this would mean another 'must'. He just sat, drank a glass of beer and then went to bed. He paused briefly to pose the question 'Why am I talking about "must" in all these situations?' His colleagues experienced exactly the opposite. For them, a 'must' was if another overnight stay was unavoidable and they could not get home.

In this Friday session, he took note of his hitherto unquestioned attitude. He had been able to question why he spoke of 'having to' go home, when his colleagues experienced it exactly the other way round. What was it about the goal of literally 'doing nothing'? So far, it had been dealt with unquestioned as 'recuperation', much deserved at the end of a long day of strenuous and stressful work. But now, he began to see it as a 'choice', which could be and needed to be explored. What was the measure of this 'must'? The colleagues seemed to follow different rules. His 'doing nothing' seemed to pull him in the direction of 'negation' while 'going/driving home' stood for life (with others).

Thinking about it conceptually, one might state that – in the background of our work – Mr A now became aware that he, in contrast to his colleagues, avoided home/the good object/breast, which they felt as a base and thus were oriented towards. Instead, he, as R. Money-Kyrle (1968) put it – and in another way D. Meltzer (1966) two years earlier – turned towards the bottom confusing it with the breast. Mentioning that he would not do something for himself, he realized the quality of his disorientation towards the anal world, in which no fertile activity can take place.

There were echoes of all this in all the sessions, but we had not yet been able to elaborate on this. The appearance of an alternative to the hitherto unquestioned issue germinated hope in the counter-transference after weeks and months of hardly any meaningful contact in the 'here and now' of the sessions. If there had been any contact, its content regularly disappeared in the subsequent 'talking over'. Now, so I thought, he had reached a decisive starting point.

Thus, I was all the more taken aback when he cancelled three sessions in the subsequent week, bit by bit, for seemingly unavoidable reasons. There had been cancellations which had to do with the expansion of the company and had not been predictable from the beginning of analysis, and these now occurred more frequently. This particular week had at last been one where he had said beforehand that he would be able to come to all four sessions, but now there was an obstruction at work which obviously came from him and which I experienced as a provocation. This pattern had given him a lot of grief in his life outside, and when we had tried to grapple with it, he had found an apt term to describe his impertinent behaviour. He said he had a stirrer (in German, *Zündler*, 'player with fire') in him, and now he was playing with fire concerning the setting. He took advantage of the Friday session but cancelled the first two sessions of the next week at short notice and spoke in the third about 'objectively' reasonable future cancellations, which made him feel uncomfortable.

I took up his discomfort and linked it with his capacity to play with fire at exactly the point where he had come into contact with essential questions. He went on to talk about appointment schedules and my having shown him how he uses them and then turned to elaborate on his theories of the stirrer. I confronted him by saying that he was now escaping with words, away from his justified unease. There was a long silence, after which he could talk more seriously and thoughtfully about something in him, which tended to 'boycott'. He talked about it in a way which conveyed how fundamental this boycott was. He described a 'peculiar mixture of resignation and triumph', which enabled me to interpret his gambling as a terrible triumph, namely, to abolish me and, in doing so, give up the part of him which sought contact (with life). That reached him.

To sum up, after he had arrived at a meaningful insight at the end of the Friday session, that had to be counteracted vehemently by enacting an exciting retreat into an anal world. Whereas during the first months, anxieties were in the foreground, now a perverse element intruded that escape.

In retrospect, I became aware that although I had questioned the higher frequency of cancellations, I had not done it each time with my usual freshness and seriousness. He often had presented the cancellations as unavoidable for business reasons, had long explanations, and so on. And I 'mistook' my not going deeply into the question each time as my attempt to not become a persecutory figure. Now I realized that with the 'solution' of not exploring it rightly, I was the disoriented one in the counter-transference. I had lost my orientation with ego judgment and let myself be disoriented by an abnormal, pathological super-ego, and malignantly twisting things. I had become an object who apparently did its job without really believing in it. Having not questioned his frequent cancellations more seriously, he experienced me (on the basis of his history) as someone not really interested in all his anxieties or responsible for him. What I had not seen clearly enough was that he now experienced me as rejecting while present – and this was what fed his anxiety.

When I put this to him, he again would respond that he 'had not thought like this' – however, the relief to be with an object, which was able again to address matters properly, was palpable. But as you will expect, it was not for long, although this and the next session were the hours of reference for the further course of his analysis. He opened one of the subsequent sessions, which followed a three-week break, with the comment that the cutter had briefly made an appearance before the session and suggested cutting – that is, missing – today's session. However, he seemed to have had a good grip on him. This was true for his appearance on that day but not for its overall effect, which he was quite aware of. This made me think later that his thought to re-train the cutter to be on his side seemed to be pointing in the right direction. Not that it would work like this, but to even entertain such an aim, that the cutter could cut the self-destructive activities, was a sign that things that had been unquestioned up to now could be thought about differently.

Next to the stirrer, the cutter was a figure 'helping' to avoid claustrophobia. But the patient had not completely lost insight about his turning away from home (in contrast to his colleagues) and what that meant. He had an idea himself of being in a topsy-turvy world and the need to reorient himself to the 'right' base.

Nevertheless, orienting activity remained difficult in the counter-transference as well. This accumulating crisis of more missed than attended sessions in the period of one month had strikingly highlighted the pull away from analysis but had not done away with the actual problems the patient experienced in a four-times-a-week setting. There were 'objective' obstacles (part of his work took him hundreds of kilometres away from home), but there was also part of him that had, as usual, responded 'No problem' to my suggestion of a four-times-a-week analysis to appear 'bigger' than what was possible/manageable for him. And now there was a new project in Austria at work, which required his presence for usually two days a week. I was involved, and there did not seem to be a right end for a cut – I needed outside help in the form of supervision to reorient myself and to enable me to make a (possibly beneficial) choice.

Issues of Choice and Orientation in Working Through Claustro-agoraphobic States

Concerning the question of choice, I would like to refer to Edna O'Shaughnessy's first publication. The then 28-year-old philosopher had dealt with the problem of 'What sort of "if" is the "if" in "I can if I choose"?' (Austin 1952, p. 125) as a contribution to a competition in the (philosophical) journal *Analysis* in 1952. O'Shaughnessy explained in the introduction that the 'if' was not one that just expressed a condition. The latter would imply that the choice was the only prerequisite needed in order that 'I can', whatever the context. She carved out a meaning in a social context in which the sentence was used in the sense of a warning, threat or reminder to be careful. The other should hear that he could not assume that I would just do this. This sentence is appropriate for un-social use. The author is obviously interested in the emotional states contained in this sentence. She showed how this could be full of spite and resentment and sensed a possible underlying sulk and other such emotions. She clarified the uncooperative use in translating 'Don't you assume I will – I may not'. The sentence is thus not used as a repudiation of an assumption but to release great emotional force in an open clash (p. 127). She talked about an 'if' in the sense of 'a possibility – in opposition'.

It opposes a 'Don't' with an 'I will, possibly'.

All this reads like a commentary on my patient and the available four sessions following the said Friday session. In this instance, I had not heard that he was possibly playing a nasty game or felt driven to play nastily. I had let myself be seduced by the manifest content (he was glad that he would be able to make all four sessions the following week) and had ignored the pull towards the unsocial, which I was familiar with. Now he reminded me forcefully, so to say, with his enacting 'Don't think that I will come – maybe I won't!' and developed a great emotional force (cf. Cuckoo 1952, p. 127). In the preceding weeks, I had occasionally attempted to establish the use or misuse of business appointments in order to undermine our endeavour here. He could verbally agree to this possibility but could not explore it further. I now had the feeling that I had underestimated the strength with which part of him wanted to drive the analysis into the wall. On one level, I had obviously taken this to be a simpler conditional – that is, if he had the possibility, he would take it. What he now confronted me with was that he could take it, but he (in part) would not.

When patients reach such a point, they frequently ask, 'Why should I do this? This does not make sense! It will harm me in the end.' Put like this, usually in an aggrieved tone. This is an expression of not-wanting-to-know. A genuine wanting-to-know would imply the pursuit of these questions and grappling with the parts of the self one would rather not have. Such questions point nevertheless in the right direction and the need to explore what hinders their pursuit of 'feeling and meaning' (cf. O'Shaughnessy 1989). On what phantasy are my patient's choices based? What object is he identified with? I felt reminded of O'Shaughnessy's paper 'Can a liar be analysed?' (1990). The key to the question about the nature of the liar is whether a version of a lying object can be experienced in the analytic situation. My patient had not lied to me directly, but still, it had come to mind. He seemed to be involved with an object which did not want to get involved, therefore, rashly agreed to everything, thus evoking the appearance of being very agreeable while actually withdrawing in this way. Thus, the analyst came into the position of acting like a claustrophobic object, being dominated by pathological projective identifications.

On one level, he experienced me in this way in the transference. I had not seriously questioned his cancellations to date, which in his experience meant that while I was giving him the appearance of a committed setting with the four sessions a week, I did not really want to or could not deal with him and did not want to be involved with him and withdrew from a deeper engagement with him. And he could identify with such an absent and rejecting object for as long as he could depend on an object which helped him experience that there was an alternative to denial, refusal, and evacuation by attempting to understand his dominant phantasy, which would leave him in an agoraphobic state.

The effect of the absence of a supportive, sustaining object was experienced in the background as a deadly threat from a present bad object, as in the case of Mr A when the first holiday break 'tripped up' his heart and made him 'stumble' emotionally and feel starved. In order to be able to think about an absence of a good object and to value this as essential for the development of one's own life, you need the experience of an object that can face the fatal consequences of its absence. Mr A's reaction had been a 'stumbling heart', and he had played down the fear of death he had experienced but had conveyed that the physical investigation, where no pathology had been found, had not sufficiently calmed him. When I made the link with my leaving him, he experienced me as an object who did not have to play down the effect of its missing. Thus, the choice was made possible with such an object, pointing to meaningful relationships with others. This had opened another perspective, which seemed to indicate that in the long run, he might be able to make a different (more beneficial) choice than the so far unquestioned one, preferring the anal world to the option of participating in the intimacy of his family. For choices to be made, the question of orientation is crucial.

When my patient had the idea that it was important for him to have the cutter on the right side, it immediately evoked an image in me. The picture implied that his vision, without adequate orientation as to what is 'right' for him, could not work for him. Our work enabled him to have a first inkling of what was 'right' – namely, not to cut off the contact with his analyst and thus withdraw into a schizoid world once more. What might be needed to cut or be limited was the pressure to 'do nothing' (or destroy things). And in the counter-transference, it needed to be understood how dependent he felt to have me on the 'right' side as an object that was not critical and demanding the impossible from him, which would have cut him off vital provisions, something that happened very easily in his experience. I also needed to register when I was threatened by resignation when he had the effect of cutting me off from all essentials, and that I would give up rather than that he would change.

Roger Money-Kyrle and, after him, Edna O'Shaughnessy, both with backgrounds in philosophy and therefore trained in thinking, made (matter-of-fact) use of the notion of orientation as a basis for the development of human thinking and symbolization (cf. Frank 2015). How can we imagine this exemplified in the development of the child? I quote O'Shaughnessy on this, who in 2006 claimed that orientation was a more important element in the psychic life than had been realized so far (p. 156).

> The finding of an object that satisfies both its emotional needs as well as its need for nourishment will transform the baby's state from one of un-integration into some sort of connectedness or integration (fragile at first) oriented towards that object. . . . As we also know, the infant oscillates between such replete, connected states and states of persecution from hunger, discomfort, delays in attention and the like. All are bad objects that threaten him with disintegration, even annihilation, which he fights by getting his good object to come to his aid. An infant who is not active in this way in both gratification and distress, an infant who is persistently passive has, I believe, suffered, and continues to suffer, some huge adversity.
>
> (2006, p. 154)

Concerning Mr A, we can assume that the mother was at times unavailable as a responsive object, thus leaving him in states of disintegration, with an annihilating quality – resulting in agoraphobia. At the same time, he could not help but identify with such an object. Her later somatic locked-in syndrome will have probably fed the terror of being trapped, being 'buried alive'. There were also other moments, a father able to care and thus moments of true understanding by the object, which was the basis for his being able to profit from my describing his conflictual states and thus strengthening an option of orientating towards a nurturing home next to the disorientation towards cutters and stirrers – figures promising salvation from all the 'musts', a universe with prevailing passivity. A lot of orientation work was needed – that is, thinking about implicitly determining unconscious phantasies in order to regain a wider range to move.

Final Notes: 'There Was a Woman Driver Who Was Driving Consistently in the Wrong Lane'

You remember we left Mr A's analysis at a point when I was in a dilemma as to how to proceed. Being drawn into a world with prevailing pathological projective identifications, I struggled with how to judge the situation. Our four-session analysis impressed as a way that had led to decisive insights and thus could help to work matters through. Would not abstaining from it mean sharing claustro-agoraphobic anxieties? On the other hand, there had been an increasing number of sessions missed for different reasons, perhaps also hinting at limits of what feels possible? Discussing these – and further – aspects in supervision helped to reorient myself: In view of the inner and outer reality, I suggested proceeding with a three-times-a-week setting for the following ten weeks and then, if appropriate, return to the four-times-a-week arrangement. (The ten weeks was the time period in which he would have been away more frequently on business.) The patient reacted with relief and was actually able to attend most of his sessions and allowed more contact with his internal world through dreams. As the period of the ten weeks came to an end, I repeatedly tried to raise the issue of how to further proceed meaningfully. His response was limited. Eventually, he told the following dream in a Friday session. Referring back to a previous dream, he said that he was once more the passenger in a car, which this time was driven by a woman – he had never dreamt this before! She was constantly veering off into the wrong lane, so he told her off to get back into the right lane. They were surrounded by threatening combine harvesters.

Mr A could not consciously find out what was appropriate for him but could dream it (to continue with me in the chosen slow lane) and thus see what filled him with overwhelming anxiety. My enquiry whether we could return to a four-times-a-week setting after the ten weeks was experienced as a dangerous veering off into the fast lane. Consciously, he was still acting in the old way ('No problem!' when I suggested four-times-a-week session), but his dream indicated that he experienced things differently.

With my patient, we saw how, in the transference and counter-transference, disorientation offered itself as 'solution' when confronted with intimacy. The struggle to recognize and differentiate the 'wrong' lane from the 'right' was one acutely suffered in the counter-transference. The nature of the object linked with questions of orientation and disorientation as an alive and interested one or one which is only apparently functioning was crucial.

We see the (unconscious) choices a patient might make from one moment to the next, which object is used to orient themselves – is he turning towards the pathological, abnormal super-ego again, or can he distance himself and attend a different orientation more actively? And in what way is the analyst affected by this? Am I capable of being sufficiently attentive to the communications of the patient? It seems important to me that we have to take it seriously when we have trouble orienting ourselves when we no longer know what the 'right' end is – then we need supervision, not as a 'miracle cure' but as an aid to enable us to think about the situation, to get reoriented (cf. Frank 2014); thus, that intimacy can be an option. While the sharpness of his claustro-agoraphobia was lessened by our work, which enabled him to feel also enjoyment when sharing intimacy with his family, the extent he could allow that for remained limited in the end.

160 Claudia Frank

Note

1 Dedicated in gratitude to Edna O'Shaughnessy.

References

Austin, J.L. (1952). Report on Analysis "Problem" No. 1. *Analysis*, *12*(6), 125–126.
Brenman Pick, I. (1995). Concern: Spurious or Real. *International Journal of Psychoanalysis*, *76*, 257–270.
Cuckoo. (1952). I Can If I Choose. *Analysis*, *12*(6), 126–128.
Frank, C. (1999). The Discovery of the Child as an Object Sui Generis of Cure and Research by Melanie Klein as Reflected in the Notes of Her First Child Analyses in Berlin 1921–1926. *Psychoanalysis and History*, 1, 155–174.
Frank, C. (2015). Zum Wurzeln der Symbolisierung in ‚sinnhaften' unbewussten Phantasien, körperlicher Erfahrungen – Der kleinianische Symbolisierungsbegriff. *Jahrbuch der Psychoanalyse*, *71*, 41–63.
Frank, C., and Böhme, I. (2014). Supervision der Supervision – Überlegungen zu einem analytischen Instrument zur Wahrnehmung und Beeinflussung von Fehlentwicklungen in der analytischen Ausbildung. *Jahrbuch der Psychoanalyse*, *69*, 157–184.
Meltzer, D. (1966). The Relation of Anal Masturbation to Projective Identification. *International Journal of Psychoanalysis*, *47*, 335–342.
Money-Kyrle, R. (1968). Cognitive Development (1978 Edition). In D. Meltzer and E. O'Shaughnessy (Eds), *The Collected Papers of Roger Money-Kyrle* (pp. 416–433). Clunie Press.
Money-Kyrle, R. (1971). The Aim of Psychoanalysis. *International Journal of Psychoanalysis*, *52*, 103–106.
O'Shaughnessy, E. (1981). A Clinical Study of a Defensive Organization. *International Journal of Psychoanalysis*, *62*, 359–369.
O'Shaughnessy, E. (1989). Seeing with Meaning and Emotion. *Journal of Child Psychotherapy*, *15*(2), 27–31.
O'Shaughnessy, E. (1990). Can a Liar be Psychoanalysed. *International Journal of Psychoanalysis*, *71*, 187–195.
O'Shaughnessy, E. (1992). Enclaves and Excursions. *International Journal of Psychoanalysis*, *73*(4), 603–611.
O'Shaughnessy, E. (1999). Relating to the Superego. *International Journal of Psychoanalysis*, *80*, 859–861.
O'Shaughnessy, E. (2006). A Conversation about Early Unintegration, Disintegration and Integration. *Journal of Child Psychotherapy*, *32*, 153–157.
Rey, H. (1979). Schizoid Phenomena in the Borderline. In J. Le Boit and A. Capponi (Eds), *Advances in the Psychotherapy of the Borderline Patient* (pp. 449–484). Jason Aronson.

Chapter 12

Claustro-Agoraphobia in Times of Covid-19

On the Problem of Making Analytic Contact When Using the Telephone and Internet for Analysis During the Coronavirus Pandemic

Kristin White

SUMMARY

During the Covid-19 pandemic crisis, telephone and internet analysis often became a temporary necessity. Kristin White, who works with German- and English-speaking patients in Berlin, shows how some patients refused to return to the normal analytic setting even when the risk of infection was very low. She assumes that these patients and some analysts, in their counter-transference, seemed to be drawn into a specific psychodynamic constellation where the remote setting offered a particular illusion in which both the fears of closeness and the fears of separation can simultaneously be defended. Largely referring to the ideas by Segal (1957), Rey (2016 [1979]), Steiner (1993), and others, White shows that under these conditions, unnoticed by patient and analyst, symbolic communication may break down, leading to a standstill in the analytic process. She describes this as a sort of psychic retreat, which becomes filled with idealised projections, whilst negative and frightening aspects of the transference situation remain split off and are deposited in the "non-telephone space". Like Henri Rey, she sees the claustro-agoraphobic dilemma as a universal condition – that is, a mode of dealing with internal and external reality which is present in us all.

TEXT

This chapter is based on my experience with telephone and internet analysis during the coronavirus epidemic. Telephone and internet analysis often became a temporary necessity during the Covid-19 pandemic, but most patients and most analysts were keen to return to in-person treatment as soon as possible when the risk of infection seemed to no longer warrant the use of the telephone and internet. However, some patients and also some analysts wanted to continue with these forms of remote analysis, even when the risk of infection had become extremely

DOI: 10.4324/9781003200284-12

low. These patients and some analysts, in their counter-transference, seemed to have been drawn into a particular psychodynamic constellation through the use of remote analysis, a constellation in which the symbolic understanding and thus the analytic work itself came to a standstill. I would like to suggest that because telephone and internet analysis offer a particular phantasy of closeness, whereas the contact is, in fact, distant or remote, there is a pull into a psychodynamic constellation in which both the fears of closeness and the fears of separation can simultaneously be defended against. It is this problematic constellation, a kind of psychic retreat, that I will attempt to describe in this chapter.

Several theoretical constructs have been helpful in the understanding of this constellation. One is Hanna Segal's thoughts on symbol formation. John Steiner's (1993) concept of the psychic retreat is also relevant, as is Henri Rey's (1994c) concept of the claustro-agoraphobia in borderline patients. Heinz Weiss (2009 and 2020 and in this book) has also described the difficulties in treating patients with claustro-agoraphobia, in particular due to their use of concrete, non-symbolic communication.

In my experience of telephone and internet analysis during the coronavirus pandemic, it was not primarily in the analysis of patients who would otherwise be diagnosed as borderline where I observed the tendency to be pulled into this psychodynamic constellation. Rather, I would suggest, with Henri Rey, that the claustro-agoraphobic position is a "universal" position into which any analysis can be pulled under certain conditions. Telephone and internet analysis seem to present one of these sets of conditions.

Because of the concrete nature of the simultaneous closeness and distance in telephone and internet analysis, this psychodynamic constellation, which Henri Rey has described as a claustro-agoraphobic and universal position, akin to the depressive or paranoid-schizoid positions described by Melanie Klein (Rey, 1994a, p. 287), perpetuates non-symbolic, concrete thinking. Thus, it becomes extremely difficult to work through or overcome this constellation in analysis.

I do not differentiate between telephone and internet analysis, although much could be said on the topic, but the differences are not relevant to the point I am trying to make in this chapter.

In communication via the telephone or the internet, the patient and the analyst are at once distant from each other, speaking from separate places and yet seeming to be very close, as the words from one person stream directly into the headset of the other. Due to the digitalisation of the words that are taken in via the telephone or the internet, there is a tendency to experience words as concrete objects rather than as symbols, words indeed, that can suddenly be broken off or disappear half-way through a sentence. I would like to suggest that the combination of actual distance and fantasised closeness in this atmosphere of concrete communication can open up a space in the transference relationship into which the analyst might also be drawn in his or her counter-transference, which becomes filled with idealised projections whilst negative aspects of the transference are split off and projected into the non-telephone space (i.e. into phantasies around returning to in-person analysis), which is then feared and rejected. The type of fears which are defended against is both the claustrophobic fears of being enclosed in the consulting room with no escape and the agoraphobic fears of separation and abandonment. These claustro-agoraphobic fears are connected to the return to in-person analysis. In practice, what we see in this situation are patients who insist that the relationship with their analyst is all good and all conflicts are resolved since embarking on telephone or internet analysis. At the same time, they resist the return to in-person analysis.

Mr A,[1] for example, was a patient who, from the beginning, had found it difficult to settle into analysis and to commit to the regularity of the sessions. He could name numerous external reasons for this: he had a second home in another country where he had grown up, and furthermore, his work demanded of him that he spend certain periods of time abroad. At the beginning of the analysis, he insisted that he needed to spend three months in another country in order to "save a relationship" in which the woman was working in another country. He mentioned that he also wanted to "test" the relationship with the woman. The analyst thought that he was actually trying to save the relationship with the analyst, as well as putting the relationship to the test, as he was deeply mistrustful of the analyst and felt unsure whether he could settle into the analytic process and whether the analyst would tolerate him with all his shortcomings. In the face of these fears, the patient put the analyst to the test in a concrete way by spending three months abroad and making her wait for him. In the years that followed, the patient was able to settle into the regularity of the sessions and was gradually able to allow the analyst to become important to him, even though he often denied her importance. He remained in the country, but the phantasy of moving away accompanied the analysis and threatened to become concrete whenever there was a longer break in the process. The analyst then interpreted the fear of the patient that he might allow himself to trust his analyst and feel needier but then be abandoned.

When the coronavirus broke out and the patient heard through the media that many workplaces were introducing the home office as the preferable mode of working, he immediately requested from his boss that he might work from home and was allowed to continue his work from home via the telephone and the internet. He then decided that if work was now going to continue online, he might as well go and stay in his second home in another country. The analyst was informed of this move only after the patient had already travelled to his second home. He had presumed that the analysis, too, would have to continue online or by telephone. His move to his second home coincided with the Easter break in the analysis, so he claimed that he had not been able to discuss the matter with his analyst. His second home was located in a remote part of the country where the internet connection was unstable, so the only way to continue the sessions was by telephone. The analyst attempted to interpret that the patient had wanted to escape the pain of feeling abandoned by the analyst during the Easter break by moving abroad, but such interpretations fell on deaf ears as the patient was only concerned with the concrete facts – it had seemed wise to travel to his second home where there had been no cases of Covid-19, and he could feel as though he were having a holiday. He was very thankful to his boss for letting him go and could not understand why the analyst seemed to have a problem with the telephone sessions. For him, it was not problematic. On the contrary, in his second home, he felt freer and happier than ever before. The fact that his boss had, in fact, only agreed to his working from home and not to him moving to another country and the fact that he had various projects and unfinished business that needed his personal attention – all this was denied. When the analyst attempted to point out the unfinished business in the analysis, the patient accused him of spoiling the beautiful relationship that had developed since they had been talking over the phone. Everything had seemed so difficult before his move. Now he felt that all his conflicts were resolved, and it was the analyst who was making things difficult by questioning his decision to move abroad.

This example shows how the space which opens up between the patient and the analyst in telephone and internet analysis functions as a kind of psychic retreat in which containment fails in the face of concrete thinking, splitting and the dominance of projective mechanisms. The patient is unable to respond to the analyst's interpretation on a symbolic level. Instead, he accuses him of spoiling the game, as it were. The "game" is one in which the patient has retreated into a place of denial, similar to the place described in John Steiner's interpretation of Oedipus at *Colonus* (1993, 116–130), a place that is conflict-free but split off from the painful internal reality of feelings of guilt, shame, and loss. Mr A also felt free of conflict as he spent his days in the beautiful nature around his second home and idealised his holiday-like feelings when he spoke to his analyst on the phone. The split-off "unfinished business" was projected into his analyst, who he felt was trying to force his negative view onto the patient, trying to make him frightened and depressed by suggesting that he was escaping a painful reality. As time went by and the analyst continued to try to understand and interpret the internal situation of the patient, the patient continued to idealise his retreat and the processes of splitting and projective identification became more entrenched. He projected all his deeper fears and conflicts into the analyst and the analytic situation. Increasingly, returning to in-person analysis thus became associated with a frightening and depressing place which the analyst was now forcing onto him.

I would like to suggest that it is, in particular, the combination of the actual distance between patient and analyst and the apparent or fantasised closeness in telephone and internet analysis, as the words of the analyst pour directly and concretely into the headset of the patient and vice versa, which tends to lead to this internal constellation with an increase in splitting and projective identification and a breakdown of the symbolic communication between the patient and the analyst. Words then become concrete objects, and the symbol is confused with the symbolised. As Hanna Segal put it,

> It struck me that concrete symbolism prevailed when projective identification was in ascendance. This also seems logical. Symbolism is a tripartite

relationship: the symbol, the object it symbolizes, and the person for whom the symbol is the symbol of the object. In the absence of a person there can be no symbol. That tripartite relationship does not hold when projective identification is in ascendance. The relevant part of the ego is identified with the object: there is not sufficient differentiation between the ego and the object itself, boundaries are lost, part of the ego is confused with the object, and the symbol which is a creation of the ego is confused with what is symbolized. It is only with the advent of the depressive position, the experience of separateness, separation and loss, that symbolic representation comes into play.

(Segal, 1991, p. 38)

When words are experienced as concrete objects in their digital internet and telephone versions, the symbol can become confused with what is symbolised, as Hanna Segal has described. Furthermore, the absence of the real person in telephone and internet analysis tends to open up a dyadic rather than a symbolic tripartite relationship. In this dyadic, undifferentiated internal state of affairs, projective identification increases and the analyst tends to actually become what the patient puts into him or her. This is very often an idealised state in which the analyst is experienced as totally supportive, totally helpful, and totally understanding and the analytic relationship is free of conflict.

It was, in fact, not just one patient who reacted to the Covid-19 outbreak in this way. Several patients moved into an idealised retreat as a result of the opportunity to move away and continue analysis at a distance on the telephone or via the internet. The important point is that it becomes almost impossible to analyse the situation. The patient feels that he has entered a perfect, undifferentiated space with his analyst. The words of the analyst are treated as concrete objects entering the patient's ear through his headset, which gives him a sense of conflict-free closeness in which all is well. This is a space in which the real distance, separation and loss are all denied, as Hanna Segal has pointed out. It is a form of psychic retreat such as that described by John Steiner – an idealised but empty world based on the denial of feelings of guilt, sadness, and helplessness. Unwanted feelings are split off and projected. The other side of this split in the analytic relationship, the "bad" relationship that is full of conflicts, is often projected into the space that is not there – that is, the relationship to the analyst in the presence of the real, whole person in the consulting room. Thus, a situation develops in which the patient fears the return to analysis in person as a dangerous and extremely threatening place.

Mr A expressed this split situation after a number of weeks in his second home by admitting to his analyst that what he would ideally like to do would be to come to her every day for sessions that were unlimited in time. But he was afraid of being honest about this wish in case she might really expect him to come back to his sessions in person rather than on the telephone, where he would then feel exposed to her scrutinising and piercing eyes that would see everything that was going on inside him. He felt that he would be caught in a prison-like space in the consulting room where the analyst had him caught in her net, and at the same time, the clock was ticking relentlessly towards the ending of the session.

Here, the split can be seen between the idealised, undifferentiated, conflict-free relationship that was experienced on the telephone and the threatening, enclosed "other" space that the consulting room had become. We know such split states from the treatment of borderline patients. John Steiner has described how it is often the eyes of the analyst that are experienced as threatening when the patient emerges from a psychic retreat (Steiner, 2011). The internal situation that was being played out in the previous example of telephone analysis can be understood in terms of what Henri Rey has termed

> claustro-agoraphobia. In this borderline state, intimacy in the psychoanalytic contact is experienced as claustrophobic: a fear of merging into the internal space of the analyst where one might be imprisoned forever. Separation from the analyst on the other hand, is experienced in an agoraphobic manner: the fear of the total loss of the self or the mind:
>
> To prevent loss of self, objects must be kept at a distance and vice versa. Thus a young schizoid man in an attempt to solve this problem would remain in his room and communicate with others by watching children play from his window and communicating with others at a distance by telephone. A woman attempted to live in my personal space by constantly walking near my residence or using the telephone to penetrate into my flat. When there was nobody there, she would let the telephone ring and fall asleep, being in my personal space. So the schizoid person, to prevent pain, anxiety or depression, splits parts of him- or herself, projects them and denies their existence. Immediately he or she experiences the opposite feelings: fear of loss, of fragmentation, and attempts to remake contact, and the vicious circle goes on.
>
> (Rey, 1994b, p. 27)

I believe that it is not merely chance that in these examples of the borderline state described by Henri Rey, it is the telephone that is the medium allowing for a simultaneous closeness to and distance from the analyst as the patient attempts to deal with his claustrophobic and his agoraphobic fears. In my experience during the Covid-19 outbreak and the ensuing telephone and internet analyses, patients are pulled into this "borderline zone", which is a latent aspect in any personality, just as psychotic elements to the personality exist in us all and can emerge when we are under extreme threat. Henri Rey, writing about these borderline states, refers to "claustro-agoraphobia and claustro-agoraphilia as a fundamental, primitive, universal 'position' (for want of a better term, and in no competition with Klein)" (Rey, 1994a, p. 287) – that is, a mode of dealing with internal and external reality which is present, if usually only latently, in us all.

Another patient, Mr B, suffered from various psychosomatic conditions, which tended to flare up in a rather alarming fashion whenever there was a break in the analysis. After the initial outbreak of the coronavirus, he asked to change to online sessions, as he felt that it was too great a risk to travel through the city, considering his weakened state of health. After the first wave of the pandemic, when most patients wanted to return to in-person psychoanalysis as soon as possible, Mr B insisted on keeping the Monday session as an online session, even though he had moved house and now lived much closer to my office. He was happy to come to his other sessions in the week in person. When I asked him why the Monday session needed to be remote, I was told that "all the offices are open on a Monday, after having been closed all weekend". I understood from this reply in concrete mode that the patient was struggling with being in the analysis during the week and out of the analysis at the weekend. He was dealing with his fears concerning the separation on Friday and the return to analysis after the weekend by keeping the Monday session in a claustro-agoraphobic mode in which he could, as it were, stand on the threshold of analysis for a day before coming back inside. Not surprisingly, the connection in these Monday sessions broke down far more regularly than usual in remote analysis. I understood this as a need on the part of the patient to break up or to split into pieces his unwanted feelings, especially of neediness and dependency.

When we change the mode of analytic communication from the direct contact in the consulting room to telephone or internet analysis, the patient and indeed the analyst can easily be pulled into a space where this claustro-agoraphobic dilemma prevails, in which both the patient and the analyst are neither in nor out of the analysis. In other words, telephone and internet analysis bring the part of the patient's internal world to the fore that in phantasy tends to retreat into a "borderland" space, not quite within and not quite without the boundaries of the psychoanalytic treatment, in the face of the simultaneous fear of being caught in the trap of the closeness in the analytic relationship and the fear of being abandoned, unable to survive emotionally alone.

In a paper discussing Rey's concept of claustro-agoraphobia, Heinz Weiss (Weiss, 2020, and see also Chapter 10 in this volume) has shown how non-symbolised, concrete thinking prevails in this state and how the non-symbolised material is projected into the analyst, distorting his or her internal space by filling it up with concrete material, so that symbolic understanding and containment in the psychoanalytic situation becomes temporarily impossible. Weiss gives an example of a patient who, while lying on the couch, conducts a long conversation on the telephone with a removal firm who is supposed to be delivering a sofa to his flat at the time of the patient's analysis session. The patient had entrusted the key to his flat to a neighbour, who had, however, not been home when the delivery men arrived. The analyst's attempt to interpret the situation symbolically in terms of the analytic situation – the fear of the patient that if he trusted that the analyst might help him, he might not be there when he needed him, as he had just experienced during the long Easter break – all this fell on deaf ears as the patient continued to fill the session and the analyst's mind with the concrete details of the problem with the delivery of the sofa.

Again, it is the telephone that upholds a situation in which the patient is simultaneously in the analysis, on the couch and at a distance from the analysis, dealing with the delivery of his sofa. The patient insists on the primary importance of the concrete information that he is giving and receiving via the telephone. The symbolic thinking that the analyst attempts to bring into the session and which can lead to a containment of the underlying fears of his patient is rejected.

All of this is very different from the containing space to which Freud was referring in his famous passage on the psychoanalytic attitude, using the telephone metaphor:

> It is easy to see upon what aim the different rules I have brought forward converge. They are all intended to create for the doctor a counterpart to the "fundamental rule of psycho-analysis" which is laid down for the patient . . . [The doctor] must turn his own unconscious like a receptive organ towards the transmitting unconscious of the patient. He must adjust himself to the patient as a telephone receiver is adjusted to the transmitting microphone. Just as the receiver converts back into sound waves the electric oscillations in the telephone line which were set up by sound waves, so the doctor's unconscious is able, from the derivatives of the unconscious which are communicated to him, to reconstruct that unconscious, which has determined the patient's free associations.
>
> (Freud, S. [1912], "Recommendations to Physicians Practising Psycho-Analysis," *The Standard Edition of the Complete Psychological Works of Sigmund Freud, Volume XII (1911–1913): The Case of Schreber, Papers on Technique and Other Works*, 115–6)

In this famous passage of Freud, the telephone is used as a metaphor for the free-floating attention of the listening analyst. In the metaphor, the analyst "must turn his own unconscious like a receptive organ towards the transmitting unconscious of the patient". The "receptive organ" is the unconscious of the analyst in his analytic attitude or stance. The analyst should "adjust himself to the patient as a telephone receiver is adjusted to the transmitting microphone". In this analytic attitude, the analyst is listening out for "the derivatives of the unconscious which are communicated to him". The keywords in all this are "as" and "like". The telephone is used as a metaphor. Working with the real telephone is a very different matter.

The trouble with the real telephone or, indeed, the internet, rather than the metaphor, is that the communication from the unconscious of the patient to the unconscious of the analyst is likely to turn into something concrete, just as the telephone itself is a concrete version of Freud's metaphor. On the telephone, we tend to listen to the real words, the real text, rather than experiencing the presence of the patient as a whole person who brings "the derivatives of the unconscious" with him into the consulting room. This leads to a potential disruption of the analytic communication.

When we put the famous words of Freud into the context of today's psychoanalytic practice, it might be tempting at first sight to think that telephone and online analysis must surely provide the perfect setting for the psychoanalytic process now that we have such high-functioning telephone and internet connections. Perhaps we never realised its advantages until we were confronted with the need for an alternative mode of communication in times of Covid-19. For years, certain psychoanalysts have been pointing out the importance of telephone and online analysis for treating patients and psychoanalytic trainees who are geographically distant from the analyst. Savege Scharff (2012) and White (2020) has given a summary of these ideas and some of the controversies around the topic. Nowadays, or so it is pointed out in the paper by Savege Scharff, we live in a globalised world, in which people travel around the world for their work and often live in different countries for periods of time, then move back to their home countries. Telephone and online analysis can offer the opportunity to continue an analysis when the patient moves away. With the telephone and internet, we can reach patients and trainees in remote parts of the country or even in other countries where they would otherwise have no access to psychoanalytic treatment or training. Surely these are all valid points. Perhaps psychoanalysis has indeed failed to move with the times and is now at last confronted with a new mode of communication which we should have accepted into our psychoanalytic practice long ago.

When psychotherapy in Berlin went online at the end of March 2020 as a reaction to the Covid-19 outbreak, this indeed was the initial reaction amongst many colleagues, trainees, and patients. Suddenly there were no more journeys to the office, to analytic treatment or to the analytic institutes. Public transport was a place of potential infection and thus to be avoided. Soon, all the schools, colleges, and universities were closed. No problem, many of us thought. We can do it all online! Teaching, training, and supervision can all go online.

All of this led to a slightly elated atmosphere. There is no doubt that this was part of a manic defence system stemmed against paranoid fears in the face of a life-threatening pandemic. And in the same, rather manic vein, schools, colleges and institutes, but also psychotherapy clinics and doctors' practices, decided to go online. The necessary technology was installed. Doctors and therapists underwent crash-course training programmes in online medicine and online treatment, and the rest was learning by doing. As analysts, we had to move fast to adapt the setting of our treatment in line with the new and ever-changing health administration regulations. Yet moving fast and learning by doing are not really compatible with psychoanalytic treatment. Rather, it is quiet contemplation and learning by experience that are the modes of analytic understanding.

As I have tried to show in this chapter, telephone and internet communication allow for a phantasy of closeness and distance simultaneously. The analyst is no longer just behind the patient's head, even though she may be there in phantasy for the patient. Instead, she is far away. As long as patient and analyst are at a safe distance from one another, the fears, the pain, and the conflicts that arise in intimacy can be avoided. Both the fears connected to closeness and the fears of separation and loss can be avoided. Instead, analysis tends to take place within the field of the patient's and, indeed, often the analyst's primitive systems of defence.

The phantasies of intimacy in remote analysis tend to be idealised, whilst the pain of separation can be split off or denied.

I think it is clear that analysis by telephone, but also internet analysis, tend to bring to the fore the non-symbolic, concrete thinking tendencies in our patients' personalities. The patients referred to in my examples were not patients who otherwise functioned primarily on a borderline level or would have been diagnosed with borderline personality disorder, even though it is clear that patients with such personality disorders will be the ones most susceptible to the problematic aspects of telephone and internet analysis described in this chapter. When remote analysis enters the claustro-agoraphobic position, the claustro-agoraphobic fears and the non-symbolic, raw material in the analytic situation become difficult or impossible to contain, as the patient and often the analyst are caught in a web of concrete thinking or the patient is unable to "hear" the interpretations on a symbolic level of understanding. Thus, the analysis tends to come to a standstill through these modes of communication. The telephone, if not understood as a metaphor, as Freud intended it, but as a concrete alternative to the actual presence of the analyst, is likely to become antagonistic to analytic understanding.

Note

1   Some details have been changed in order to protect the identity of the patient.

References

Freud, S. (1912). Recommendations to Physicians Practising Psycho-Analysis. In *SE* (Vol. 12). Hogarth Press.

Rey, H. (1994a). Awake, Going to Sleep, Dreaming, Awaking, Awake: Comments on W. Clifford M. Scott. Rey, H. In *Universals of Psychoanalysis in the Treatment of Psychotic and Borderline States* (pp. 277–287). Free Association Books.

Rey, H. (1994b). The Schizoid Mode of Being and the Space-Time Continuum (Before Metaphor). In *Universals of Psychoanalysis in the Treatment of Psychotic and Borderline states* (pp. 7–30). Free Association Books.

Rey, H. (1994c). *Universals of Psychoanalysis in the Treatment of Psychotic and Borderline states*. Free Association Books.

Rey, J.H. (2016 [1979]). Schizoid Phenomena in Borderline Syndrome. In: Bott-Spillius, E. (ed.), *Melanie Klein Today. Developments in Theory and Practice* (Vol. 1, 5th edition, 253–287). Klett-Cotta.

Savege Scharff, J. (2012). Clinical Issues in Analyses Over the Telephone and Internet. *International Journal of Psychoanalysis*, *93*, 81–95.

Segal, H. (1957). Notes on Symbol Formation. *International Journal of Psychoanalysis*, *38*, 391–397.

Segal, H. (1991). *Dream Phantasy and Art*. Routledge.

Steiner, J. (1993). *Psychic Retreats*. Routledge.

Steiner, J. (2011). *Seeing and Being Seen*. Routledge.

Weiss, H. (2009). Das Labyrinth der Borderline-Kommunikation. In *Klinische Zugänge zum Erleben von Raum und Zeit*. Klett-Cotta.

Weiss, H. (2020). Claustro-Agoraphobia: The impact of concrete thinking on the analyst's internal space. Published in German: Weiss, H. (2020). Das agora-claustrophobe Dilemma des Borderline-Patienten – behandlungstechnische Herausforderungen. *Zeitschrift für Individualpsychologie*, *45*, 188–203.

White, K. (2020). Practising as an Analyst in Berlin in Times of the Coronavirus: The Core Components of Psychoanalytic Work and the Problem of Virtual Reality. *International Journal of Psychoanalysis*, *101*, 580–584.

Conclusion

Susan Finkelstein

It is important to recognize that although claustro-agoraphobia is a fairly recent subject of psychoanalytic attention, it has been with us for thousands of years – the proof is the vivid depictions that have been handed down to us by philosophers, poets, and writers over many generations and from many cultures. Psychoanalysis has always drawn powerfully on ancient literary and cultural traditions.

In fact, "Know thyself," the aphorism inscribed over the entrance of the Temple of Apollo at Delphi, is perhaps the most concise expression available to us of the philosophy that ultimately became psychoanalysis. Sigmund Freud exemplified it as he scrutinized himself – his dreams, his phantasies, his sexual desires, and less predictably his apparently irrational instincts, guilts, terrors, and aggressions. He represented psychoanalysis as a science and offered a copious body of theories and case studies to support that contention, which even now is by no means universally accepted. But since long before Freud began developing his ideas, science or not, into a structured discipline, people have relied on philosophers, artists, and playwrights for insight into human nature. It is true that psychoanalysis elaborated upon what these humanists, some of them ancient indeed, already knew, but it is also true that the wisdom in their work informed it from its inception and illustrates its worth now, both to psychoanalytic thinkers and to their skeptical contemporaries.

In a powerful image of Western literature, Plato (*The Republic*, Book 7) describes a group of persons imprisoned in a cave, chained so that they can see only the shadows cast upon them. They interpret this as the only reality they have ever known. Plato then imagines what might happen should a prisoner escape from their cave and bear witness to another reality, unrepresented and unexperienced by him. The Parable of the Cave depicts the dread of living with uncertainty about safety and danger, knowledge and ignorance, of time itself stopping, of the terror of not knowing where we end and the world begins (Finkelstein 2016). These are universal human concerns that have fascinated psychoanalysts since Freud discovered the science at the dawn of the twentieth century.

These cave dwellers, often referred to as living in psychic retreats (Steiner, Chapter 8), were living in what Henri Rey coined the *claustro-agoraphobic dilemma* (Rey, Chapter 7). Rey characterizes the intense claustrophobic anxiety of being trapped inside the metaphorical cave, which he states in phantasy represents the mother's womb and the agoraphobic anxiety of expulsion from it. Individuals suffering from claustro-agoraphobic anxieties fear imprisonment inside or outside of their objects. Claustrophobic fears of suffocation exist while inside the womb; agoraphobic terror of loss of self or other overwhelms while outside. The permeable boundary of where the self ends and the other begins can lead to ego regression, decompensation, and even madness. These combined inside-outside annihilation anxieties leave the claustro-agoraphobe feeling desperate, with no place of safety: "There is nowhere for the claustro-agoraphobic" (Rey). The phantasy of living inside the mother's body leaves the individual unable to distinguish between self and other, inside and outside, psychic and external reality. This results in an illusion of omnipotence and omniscience and inability to trust or depend on others.

Henri Rey depicts "marsupial space" as an ideal maternal environment (container) for holding and containing the negotiation of in-between spaces – inside-outside spaces for the individual to develop physically and emotionally within the security of the baby-mother dyad. This concept applies to the psychoanalytic patient-analyst dyad, which has the potential for emotional containment that was unavailable in the early emotional development of the child-mother dyad. Heinz Weiss (Chapter 10) describes the flooding of the analyst's mind by the patient's projective identifications, preventing the formation of a marsupial space for containment. He explains that this environment can improve once the patient is able to move from concrete thinking to symbolization. With this progress, the reparative function of the psychoanalyst can convert the one-dimensional space to the necessary marsupial space of the patient-analyst dyad for emotional thinking and growth to occur.

Rey expands Melanie Klein's concept of psychic reparation to the claustro-agoraphobe's terror of doing damage to the mother while inside her womb or to her and others while outside of confinement (Rey). Examples from literary references of this dilemma and the dread of doing damage to oneself and one's internal objects will be discussed shortly.

In addition to Plato, more recent authors have also been fascinated by imprisonment and the terrors of its claustro-agoraphobic implications and have been inspired to create powerful and menacing visions of it. One of the best known is Edgar Allan Poe's "The Pit and the Pendulum" (1842), in which a prisoner sentenced to death by the Inquisition contemplates his fate from his cell. First, he discovers a deep pit at the center of his dungeon, from which he is saved by chance. Later, strapped to a board by his captors, he is terrified to see the scythe of Father Time swinging down from the ceiling, coming closer and closer to his body. He escapes this threat, too, this time by his own ingenuity, only to discover that the walls of the cell have become red-hot and are closing in on him, driving him back towards the very pit he had managed to avoid earlier. In Poe's story, however, there is no internal work of escape. This prisoner's eventual last-minute rescue comes from outside, as an enemy army conquers the Inquisition and its torturers.

Perhaps it is Franz Kafka (1883–1924) who, among modern authors, best depicts the claustro-agoraphobic agonies of a life trapped between the terror of a self-imposed prison and the terror of leaving it. Kafka's absurdist novels and stories portray tortured souls who struggle with identity, alienation, self-hatred, and the dilemma we depict in this book – the conflict between the wish to free themselves from their imprisonment and the fear that there is either something dangerous or nothing meaningful outside it.

In *The Metamorphosis* (1915), Kafka's protagonist Gregor Samsa awakens to find himself transformed into a huge insect. His small room is a refuge, but it is also a prison and an experience of hell because it is his only alternative – now that he is no longer human, there is no "outside" space that one such as Gregor can seek. His relationships with the people who once mattered to him dissolve; he is "vermin," an object of disgust and contempt to them.

It is hard not to wonder to what extent this was Kafka's own experience – feeling like a revolting alien, hated by others and by himself. He was engaged twice to a beloved fiancée, but he could never bring himself to marry her (*Letters to Felice*, 1973). In "The Burrow" (1924), his last story (unfinished) before he died from tuberculosis at age 42, the protagonist is another trapped animal, a mole-like creature, who constructs endless tunnels in which to hide, always looking to keep himself safe from attack by enemies whom he does not recognize as internal. Like other claustro-agoraphobes, Kafka could not live securely inside his own body or feel safe enough in a relationship to share someone else's. His world was one of bodily and spiritual suffering. In the dark underground existences he imagined, he portrayed his personal struggles and his search for meaning, but also his ultimate sense of powerlessness. To this day, his writing vividly conveys the extremes of anxiety, desperation, and alienation that cause people to search for safety in metaphorical caves and burrows and also the recognition that the only safety within such entombment is illusory.

Kafka's moles living in underground tunnels may have an illusory protection, but they are alone. Kafka's "in-betweenness" of loving and hating himself and Felice and self-contempt and accusations consigned him to isolation. Poe's claustrophobic walls and terrors of the outside were suffocating and crushing. The omnipotence of living in internal structures provides some illusory structure but, as Mason reminds us, also "produces panic and explosion, in a desperate attempt to escape, even at the cost of disintegration. The internal effect of the omniscient suffocating super-ego could be likened to an attack of acute claustrophobia of the mind" (1981, p. 143).

Samuel Beckett in *Not I* (2014 [1972]) and *Endgame* (2014 [1957]) depicts a symbolic twentieth-century hell, a claustrophobic prison in which there can be no escape either from the world of one's own making or from the world that others have made. In his short poem "Neither," Beckett charts the shadowy movement "from impenetrable self to impenetrable unself/by way of neither" (2014 [1979]).

Long before Freud began developing his ideas about the mind into a structured discipline, people have relied on philosophers, poets, and playwrights and their interpretation of mythology for insight into human nature. It is true that psychoanalysis has made eager use of what these giants already knew, repeatedly elaborating and building upon them, but it is also true that the wisdom in their work and the clarity of their vision also offer powerful illustrations of sometimes arcane-seeming psychoanalytic concepts, both to analysts and to their skeptical contemporaries. The best-known example of this process and the symbiosis between psychoanalysis and literature is the well-known and controversial Oedipus complex. Freud was clearly inspired by the insights in Sophocles' fifth-century-BC tragedy *Oedipus Rex*. He commented to Wilhelm Fliess that "the Greek legend seizes upon a compulsion which everyone recognizes because he senses its existence within himself. Everyone in the audience was once a budding Oedipus in fantasy and each recoils in horror from the dream fulfillment here transplanted into reality" (Freud, Letter to Fliess, October 15, 1897, p. 272). Certainly, Freud was not alone in his appreciation; we all owe a debt to Sophocles for his telling of one man's torturous encounter with his own truth. But for Freud, the Oedipus complex was more than that; it was psychological bedrock, integrating as it did present culture with the history of civilization and encapsulating the essential human struggle to come to terms with the pains of conscious awareness and the terrors of knowledge and the unconscious.

More than a century after Freud's breakthrough, psychoanalysts are still using that myth as a source of inspiration and instruction. Having learned at last who his parents were, how they abandoned and tried to kill him, and what that meant for his own marriage and progeny, Oedipus is ravaged by the guilt that leads to his self-blinding and the suicide of Jocasta, his mother and wife. This story suggests more than the specific universal emotional experience on which Freud focused. It is also a cautionary tale about the potential dangers of reality and the emotional challenges of situations that one may unconsciously suspect but not consciously accept. Oedipus's struggle is not only the classic illustration (for psychoanalysts and others) of a particular emotional conflict but also a dramatic depiction of the danger of knowing. As such, it is a reminder to psychoanalysts of Freud's argument that psychoanalysis is by definition a perilous process.

The psychoanalytic process requires courage: courage to give up psychic retreats and hiding places, to confront frightening truths and primitive anxieties, and to face the fear and the fact of our capacity for harm. Unlike an analytic patient, of course, Oedipus had no mother to help him learn to contain his emotional torments and manage his guilts as a child and no analyst to help him work through them later. These are very difficult jobs, as Sophocles shows us clearly, and as analysts, we need to be aware that they remain difficult jobs for our claustro-agoraphobic patients. The acquisition of knowledge and the fulfillment of desire confront us with complex realities, which may include our own responsibility for damaged internal and external relationships.

Even before the Greeks, legend provided insight into the human condition and the psychoanalytic journey that it later inspired. The Mesopotamian *Epic of Gilgamesh* (circa 2000 BC) is the oldest known Babylonian text. Etched in cuneiform in clay tablets and translated in the mid-1870s by George Smith, it predates Hesiod and Homer, the earliest known Greek poets, by at least a thousand years (*The Epic of Gilgamesh*, trans. George, "Introduction," p. xxiii). *Gilgamesh* is a complex story about the fear of death and the search for immortality and meaning. Like Sophocles' play, it is not only a work of art but also a vivid portrayal of important psychological aspects of human growth.

Gilgamesh is a demigod who behaves toward his elders and his community with tyrannical disregard. The elders give him a mortal friend named Enkidu for companionship and to calm his arrogant ways. While journeying together, the two insult and offend the gods, who punish them by sentencing Enkidu to death. Gilgamesh is grief-stricken. He cannot accept his companion's death or the fact of death itself, and he falls into a melancholic identification with his deceased friend. At first, his response is to set off on a quest for immortality, but as Gilgamesh matures (in part through his dependence on the help of others), he becomes able to mourn his friend's death and accept the facts of mortality, his own limitations, and his responsibility for his arrogant disregard of the gods that contributed to the death of Enkidu. His journey calms his manic behavior and grandiose expectations. He learns to acknowledge the worth of his own contributions, specifically the construction of walls that protect his city and the hope that his "tale" will endure. These changes indicate Gilgamesh's capacity to mourn, accept reality and responsibility, forgive himself, and work toward the reparation of his damaged objects. These are requisite to emerging from the claustro-agoraphobic dilemma.

Claustro-agoraphobic patients seeking therapy are mostly unaware of their internal worlds and the situation their defenses have kept them entrapped in. They cannot live comfortably inside or outside of the relationship. They need an analyst to help them mourn, to lessen their primitive super-ego, to work through their guilts and shames, and to make reparation to those whom they have damaged in actuality or in phantasy. The analytic experience and relationship create the potential for a new space for reflection, growth, and change – a space in which the work of reparation can be done.

Just as the Greek dramatists used their choruses as participants/observers pointing out the dangers of both knowledge and denial, so do psychoanalysts and patients participate in and observe the scenarios of conflict and growth that emerge in their work together. Plato's cave dwellers and Kafka's moles do not have the freedom of safety living inside their minds or inside the minds of others. For metaphorical cave dwellers, the analytic space can be an alternative area and means of freedom from entrapment inside the mother's body and the retrieval of projective identifications that leave the individual depleted and alone.

The claustro-agoraphobic dilemma has been around for millennia, although the concept was not named by Rey until 1979. Our newer clinical awareness of its manifestations will deepen modern appreciation of older works of art and philosophy. It is worth recognizing how profoundly those older works have contributed to the new awareness that we have been outlining in this book. It is one more way that psychoanalysis will enrich and expand the psychoanalytic worldview – if we listen and pay attention.

References

Beckett, S. (2014 [1957]). Endgame. In *The Collected Poems of Samuel Beckett*. Grove Press.
Beckett, S. (2014 [1972]). Not I. In *The Collected Poems of Samuel Beckett*. Grove Press.
Beckett, S. (2014 [1979]). Neither. In *The Collected Poems of Samuel Beckett*. Grove Press.
Finkelstein, S.N. (2016). Psychosomatic Illness in a Claustro-Agoraphobic Patient. In P. Sloate (Ed.), *From Soma to Symbol* (pp. 173–196). Karnac.
Freud, S. (1897). October 27, 1897. In J.M. Masson (Ed. and Trans.) *The Complete Letters of Sigmund Freud to Wilhelm Fliess 1887–1904* (1985) (p. 272). Belknap Press of Harvard University Press.
George, A. (1999). Introduction. In *The Epic of Gilgamesh* (A. George, Trans). Penguin Books. p. XXIII. Penguin Books.
Kafka, F. (1996 [1915]). *The Metamorphosis and Other Stories*. Dover.
Kafka, F. (1931 [1946]). *The Burrow*. Schocken Books.
Kafka, F. (1973). *Letters to Felice* (E. Heller and J. Born, Eds). Schocken Books.
Mason, A. (1981). Do I Dare Disturb the Universe? A Memorial to W.R. Bion. In J. Grostein (Ed.), *The Suffocating Superego: Psychotic Break and Claustrophobia* (pp. 140–165). Karnac.
Plato. (1991). *The Republic. Book VII* (A. Bloom, Trans., pp. 193–220). Basic Books.
Poe, E.A. (2009 [1842]). *The Pit and the Pendulum*. Penguin.

Index

Page numbers in *italics* indicate figures.

For Product Safety Concerns and Information please contact our EU
representative GPSR@taylorandfrancis.com
Taylor & Francis Verlag GmbH, Kaufingerstraße 24, 80331 München, Germany